Cambridge Studies in Medical Anthropology

Editor

ALAN HARWOOD *University of Massachusetts, Boston*

Editorial Board

WILLIAM DRESSLER *University of Alabama*
RONALD FRANKENBERG *Brunel University, UK*
MARY JO GOOD *Harvard University*
SHARON KAUFMAN *University of California, San Francisco*
SHIRLEY LINDENBAUM *City University of New York*
MARGARET LOCK *McGill University*
CATHERINE PANTER-BRICK *University of Durham, UK*

Medical anthropology is the fastest growing specialist area within anthropology, both in North America and in Europe. Beginning as an applied field serving public health specialists, medical anthropology now provides a significant forum for many of the most urgent debates in anthropology and the humanities. It includes the study of medical institutions and health care in a variety of rich and poor societies, the investigation of the cultural construction of illness, and the analysis of ideas about the body, birth, maturity, ageing, and death.

This series includes theoretically innovative monographs, state-of-the-art collections of essays on current issues, and short books introducing main themes in the subdiscipline.

1. Lynn M. Morgan, *Community Participation in Health: The Politics of Primary Care in Costa Rica*
2. Thomas J. Csordas (ed.), *Embodiment and Experience: The Existential Ground of Culture and Health*
3. Paul Brodwin, *Medicine and Morality in Haiti: The Contest for Healing Power*
4. Susan Reynolds Whyte, *Questioning Misfortune: The Pragmatics of Uncertainty in Eastern Uganda*
5. Margaret Lock and Patricia Kaufert, *Pragmatic Women and Body Politics*
6. Vincanne Adams, *Doctors for Democracy*
7. Elisabeth Hsu, *The Transmission of Chinese Medicine*
8. Margaret Lock, Allan Young and Alberto Cambrosio (eds.), *Living and Working with the New Medical Technologies: Intersections of Inquiry*

Further titles will include:
Susan Reynolds Whyte, Sjaak van der Geest and Anita Hardon, *The Social Lives of Medicines*
James Trostle, *Epidemiology and Culture*

Meaning, Medicine, and the "Placebo Effect"

n
gs
h
ly
f-
ts
"

s,
l-
:r
d

-
e
-
n
e

Meaning, Medicine, and the "Placebo Effect"

Daniel E. Moerman

University of Michigan-Dearborn

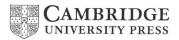
CAMBRIDGE
UNIVERSITY PRESS

PUBLISHED BY THE PRESS SYNDICATE OF THE UNIVERSITY OF CAMBRIDGE
The Pitt Building, Trumpington Street, Cambridge, United Kingdom

CAMBRIDGE UNIVERSITY PRESS
The Edinburgh Building, Cambridge CB2 2RU, UK
40 West 20th Street, New York, NY 10011-4211, USA
477 Williamstown Road, Port Melbourne, VIC 3207, Australia
Ruiz de Alarcón 13, 28014 Madrid, Spain
Dock House, The Waterfront, Cape Town 8001, South Africa

http://www.cambridge.org

First published 2002

Printed in the United Kingdom at the University Press, Cambridge

Typeface Plantin 10/12 pt   *System* LaTeX 2$_\varepsilon$ [TB]

A catalogue record for this book is available from the British Library

ISBN 0 521 80630 5 hardback
ISBN 0 521 00087 4 paperback

For Claudine,
with admiration, affection, and love

Contents

Figures

Tables

Acknowledgments

I wrote my first scholarly article about issues discussed in this book in 1979. I have, then, worked on and thought about the matter for about twenty-five years. The University of Michigan-Dearborn has been my professional home for that entire period; I owe a great debt to colleagues – both faculty, staff and administrators – who, in that time, have supported me intellectually and institutionally. Among them are Victor Wong, Jim Foster, John Presley, Paul Wong, Robert Simpson, and Dan Little, all administrators who have strongly supported the principle of the teacher-scholar which created the opportunity for the work. Drew Buchanan provided invaluable technical and personal support; Bob Fraser provided those, plus helpful counsel on biblical translations. Department chairs Don Levin, Rick Straub and Barry Bogin provided ample real support in time, equipment, and space for my various efforts. Many colleagues, too, helped by reading chapters or the whole text, or by engaging in discussion about both the larger and the smaller issues one confronts in such work. Among those who were particularly helpful were Paul Zitzewitz, John Gillespie, Dan Swift, Barry Bogin, and Katie Anderson-Levitt. In a class by himself is Larry Radine who helped me over what seemed at the time to be an insurmountable obstacle; thanks, Larry. Colleagues from around the US and Europe also helped in many ways: Bob Ader, Mirielle Belloni, Steve Bolling, Loring Brace, Howard Brody, Claire Cassidy, Nicholas Christakis, Tom Csordas, Ton de Craen, Susan DiGiacomo, Linda Engel, Michel Gabrielli, Rick Gracely, Harry Guess, Robert Hahn, Ellen Idler, Wayne Jonas, Ted Kaptchuk, Irving Kirsch, Martin Leon, Claude Levi-Strauss, Shirley Lindenbaum, Margaret Lock, Bruce Moseley, John Payer, Lola Romanucci-Ross, John Ross, Pat Rozee, Bill Stebbins, Jon Stoessl, Sjaak van der Geest, and Andrew Vickers all helped in one way or the other, large or small, sometimes not really knowing that our conversations were going to end up here (I may not have known it at the time either). Bill McGrew provided the photo of "chimpanzee dentistry," and also was a valuable advisor on other matters regarding primates. Although it didn't start until the book was half done, the "Placebo Group," organized by Anne Harrington as part of the program of the Harvard University Mind/Brain/Behavior Initiative, has been enormously influential in my final shaping of this work. The broadly interdisciplinary discussions with that group are among the very finest academic experiences I have ever had; thanks to Anne Harrington, Nick Humphrey, Howard Fields, Fabrizio Benedetti, Jamie Pennebaker, Dan Wegner and Ginger Hoffman. Alan Harwood suggested the project, and shepherded it along with gentle but persistent pressure for the best book I could produce. My sister-in-law – a very fine scientist – Elena Moerman, and my old friend and neighbor Will Cummings read all or most of the manuscript and made many valuable suggestions. Good friends Jan Berry and John Copley provided deeply appreciated neighborly support. Most long suffering perhaps have been the hundreds of students in Anthro 430 Medical Anthropology over the years who have heard these arguments and helped me to make them both clear and persuasive. The National Science Foundation generously supported some of the work described here; Stuart Plattner of NSF was particularly helpful to me on many occasions.

Finally, my family – my wife Claudine, our children and their spouses Jennifer, Chris, Fred, Patti, Anne, and grandchildren Allison and Spencer – have all heard this, too, and have kept me smiling.

I have had great fun with this project; I kept telling myself how easy it would be to write a "placebo book" because it doesn't have anything in it.

Introduction: "Pickle ash" and "high blood"

My first introduction to something that might be called "medical anthropology" occurred in 1969, although at the time, I had never heard that phrase. I was doing fieldwork on St. Helena Island in South Carolina as part of my Ph.D. work. St. Helena is a barrier island, just across the Broad River to the north from much better known Hilton Head Island. Interested in family organization in a black community (debates raged in the 1960s about "the black family"), I thought that a thorough investigation of such families in a real community would be worthwhile. As I pursued my genealogies and spoke with these kind people, I heard an occasional reference to the use of certain plants – they called them "weeds" – to treat various illnesses. Intrigued, I pursued the matter, and found a number of people eager to talk about it. Eventually, I was able to identify three dozen or so "weeds" that were part of everyday use; most were better known to older than younger Islanders, but most everyone knew something about it. The whole matter seemed very odd to me; today, surrounded by "health food" and "natural medicine" shops, with everyone taking Echinacea to stimulate his or her immune system, and Gingko to ward off Alzheimer's disease, it doesn't seem so unusual to hear about medicinal plants, but in the 1960s, it was odd indeed. I wondered if anyone else had ever used those plants for anything, and did they work? I can't tell that story here, even though the answers to these questions deeply inform my understandings of what I *will* write about. I have written a good deal about those issues, however, and some of it is readily available (see, for example, Moerman 1982, 1989, 1998b).

Some of this botanical medicine seemed quite empirical. The bark of a tree known as prickly ash (*Zanthoxylum americanum* or perhaps *Z. clava-herculis*) was reputedly a powerful treatment for diarrhea in pigs. Actually, what I was told was more colorful than this. One older gentleman said that the "pickle ash" would "check up run stomach in pigs," but that you had to be careful not to give them too much or you might "cork 'em for keeps!" These two species of plants, *Z. clava-herculis* (Hercules' club) and *Z. americanum* (prickly ash), were part of professional American medicine

1

for at least a century and were listed in the US Pharmacopoeia from 1820 until about 1930, when they were replaced with other, newer drugs.

But there were other aspects of this medical system which did not overlap with Western medicine. On the one hand, there was no talk about "germs," or "viruses," or even "stress." And nothing about avoiding sitting in drafts. But, for some reason, babies (my year-old daughter was with us in South Carolina) should never go outside without a hat on, even in the midst of a blazing August summer day. I'm still not sure why, but it seemed as if some kind of wraiths or spirits could enter the baby's head; I'm not sure people were really clear on just why this was the correct thing to do, but they got quite upset if I didn't put a hat on Jennifer. Then again, people from Kansas or Wisconsin usually aren't too clear on why you can "catch a cold" (a viral infection) after sitting in a draft or getting your feet wet. Regardless of whether it was all worked out logically, it was clear that these people had a very different understanding of illness than I did.

The most interesting aspect of this belief system involved the idea of a dichotomy in the body's "pressure." There was a constellation of symptoms which were due to the fact that the pressure of the body was too high: for example, childhood fevers, adult colds, and an illness typically experienced by older people characterized by nausea, dizziness, short memory and headache called "high blood." There was also an opposite condition, for which I never learned a distinctive name but which might have resembled "spring fever," characterized by weakness, lassitude, constipation, and, perhaps, something like depression.

The pressure in the body was considered to be a function of the blood. If the blood were too "sweet," your pressure would rise and you would get a fever or, perhaps, high blood. Note that this wasn't simply "blood pressure," but a more pervasive, generalized pressure. The blood could get sweet for several reasons, but the typical explanation was dietary: people tended, they said, to eat too much meat, sweets, and grease. The treatment for this problem involved taking medicines which would "bitter the blood." Typical medicines for this were the root of the coral bean (*Erythrina herbacea*), garlic (*Allium ampeloprasum*), life everlasting (*Pseudognaphalium obtusifolium*), horse nettle (*Solanum carolinense*), and Virginia snakeroot (*Aristolochia serpentaria*). The less common low blood conditions were treated with sweet medicines like sassafras (*Sassafras albidum*), carrot seeds (from Queen Anne's Lace, *Daucus carota*), sugar, and wine.

Although this African-American understanding of health and illness has been described in some detail since then (Snow 1993), at the time I had not heard of it. It seemed vaguely similar to the hot/cold systems of Latin America, but only in its form, not its content. Thus, there were two poles, but it was not a comprehensive classification of objects, with each food being labeled "sweet" or "bitter." Regardless, as I thought about it more, I began to wonder what effect such a set of understandings and beliefs might have had on the actual healing processes in this community. It didn't take long for me to learn that, indeed, the "weeds" they were using were effective medications; what about the ideas they used as they mobilized their medicines? Did these make any difference?

I had been very broadly trained as a graduate student in anthropology; I didn't think of myself as a cultural anthropologist, or a biological anthropologist, but as what I called an "unhyphenated anthropologist" (with an ironic tip of the hat to Barry Goldwater, for readers old enough to remember). To me, a human being was simultaneously a biological and a cultural creature; biology and culture were, for me, the warp and woof of the human fabric. The clearest cases were evolutionary: the reduction of the size of the human dentition which accompanied the dramatic expansion of material culture over a million or more years; the apparent relationship between evolving neurology (evident in brain expansion) over the time of the unambiguous development of a symbolic culture in the past 100,000 years; and so on. But these things happened a long time ago, were hard to see, bedeviled with dating problems, and intensely controversial. I was eager to find a situation in which it was plausible to investigate the ways in which cultural and symbolic processes interacted with biological ones, in real time.

I stumbled on the placebo effect sometime in the mid-1970s. I don't remember just how. But it quickly became apparent to me that there were important anthropological possibilities in this topic. My first published paper on the matter was titled "The Anthropology of Symbolic Healing" (Moerman 1979). Although that paper discussed the meaningful quality of surgery, it wasn't until a bit later that I discovered placebo heart surgery, which became the center of my paper "Physiology and Symbols" (Moerman 1983). By then, as the title indicates, I had realized how important (and how utterly difficult) it was to avoid reductionism, to avoid the trap of sociobiological, or even evolutionary, determinism, in the analysis of health and healing. While it seemed clear to me that people who could respond positively to medical ritual or meaning might have an evolutionary advantage over their fellows who did not, I was very chary of an approach which found any odd institution or behavior explained as a device to enhance an individual's fitness or the inclusive fitness (the evolutionary success – the increased fertility – of an individual's close relatives). During the height of the Vietnam war, it seemed folly to me to think this way; I simply couldn't imagine any way that, say, 370,000 combat deaths in the American Civil War could enhance anyone's fitness, inclusive or otherwise.

The challenge became one of persistently trying to avoid "privileging" either biological or meaningful processes while simultaneously avoiding the simplistic dualism of "mind vs. body". As you will see later on, the process of thinking about your own pain – whether a banged shin or sprained ankle – can enhance or diminish the pain. The two elements are aspects of the same process.

This book, then, focuses on the problem of understanding what is commonly called the "placebo effect." I will argue that this is an unfortunate term, used carelessly for such a broad range of phenomena that we should probably abandon it; or, if we must keep it, we should use it only to refer to the changes observed in the subjects in a control group in an experiment. Many of those changes need have no relationship at all to those dimensions of human life which are simultaneously cultural and biological. And I will attempt to tease out of that heterogenous mass of phenomena the ones which engage the biological consequences of experiencing knowledge, symbol, and meaning. I will call those things the "meaning response." But I will argue as well that many more complex aspects of life work in essentially the same way for all human beings, and that many kinds of meaningful events in our lives – medical or otherwise – affect us for good or ill. And I will propose a general way of thinking about these issues and researching them.

A plan of the book

The book is in three parts. Part I describes the meaning response carefully. Part II outlines some applications, objections, and opportunities. Part III includes some broad conclusions regarding the relationship between meaning and biology.

Part I begins with a discussion of sickness and healing. Chapters 1 and 2 describe some of the factors involved in getting well. Chapter 3 describes some of the techniques used by researchers to sort out just what parts of a healing intervention can be attributed to different elements of it; this chapter shows how we can see placebo effects in a clinical trial, and why it is harder to see them as clearly in non-Western medical systems. Chapters 4, 5, and 6 consider the various factors which shape and moderate medical interventions. Chapter 4 focuses on relationships, especially between doctors and patients. Chapter 5 focuses on *formal* factors, such as the shape, color, and amounts of medicines, and reviews the meaning of surgery. Chapter 6 looks at more systematic sorts of knowledge which follow from cultural differences among peoples, and how they affect both illness and healing. Throughout, I develop the idea that the most important element in these factors, their underlying common factor, is "meaning."

Part II considers some applications of the idea of the meaning response. In Chapter 7, I review the field of psychotherapy and psychiatric medicine where the manipulation of meaning – in "talking cures," for example – is most evident and obvious. In Chapter 8, I review the neurobiology and cultural biology of pain; this area has the clearest and most complete experimental and cultural evidence for the role of meaning in medicine. In Chapter 9, I review two complex areas where much more needs to be researched, but where one can make plausible hypotheses about meaning and the significant improvement of human health; these areas, usually not thought of in this context, show how powerful the meaning response is as a way to understand health and healing. Chapter 10 addresses two other widely held theoretical approaches to placebo effects – conditioning theory and expectancy theory – and explains why I believe the approach through meaning is preferable. Chapter 11 addresses ethical issues which many have raised about the placebo effect and suggests an approach to dealing with them.

Part III, made up of the final two chapters, includes a synthetic account of these human biological processes. It suggests a model for understanding when they will, and when they will not, occur, and in particular why it is so hard to convince people about the validity of these notions which are, at one level or another, quite obvious – as obvious as the fact that you might smile when you see a puppy, or cry at a sad movie.

Although the use of inert medications, "placebos," can inform us about many fascinating aspects of human cultural and biological life, I hope that a close reader of this book will see that it is not really about the placebo effect. It is about the interaction of biology and meaning in human life (which accounts for portions of what is usually called the placebo effect.) Human beings are uniquely "cultural animals." That phrase is, on its face, an oxymoron, a contradiction in terms. But close consideration shows that what we think, say, and know about the world can have a dramatic influence on our biology, as culture and biology overlap in powerful and important ways.

Part I

The meaning response

1   Healing and medical treatment

> Ever since [ship physician] Stephen Maturin had grown rich with their
> first prize [about 1790] he had constantly laid in great quantities of
> asafetida, castoreum and other substances, to make his medicines more
> revolting in taste, smell and texture than any others in the fleet; and he
> found it answered – his hardy patients *knew* with their entire beings that
> they were being physicked.
>
> Patrick O'Brian, *Master and Commander*, 1970

Even fictional doctors know that their patient's attitudes and understanding of medicine and treatment are a fundamental part of the healing
process.

An ulcer trial

In the early 1990s, Dr. Frank Lanza, a gastroenterologist from Houston,
Texas, led a large team of doctors in a test of a new drug for treating ulcers.
Over 300 people participated in the trial which compared the effectiveness
of a new drug known as lansoprazole (its trade name is "Prevacid") with
another, older, drug for ulcers called ranitidine ("Zantac"). The people
who entered this study were diagnosed with ulcers by having a procedure
called an *endoscopy*. In this procedure, a fiber optic tube – an endoscope –
is put down the patient's esophagus, and a technician examines the wall of
the gut on a little television screen. In each case, only after the technician
saw an ulcer in the patient's stomach was the person admitted to the study.

After this diagnosis, patients were randomly assigned to one of several
groups. Some patients got Zantac (300 mg), some got Prevacid (15 mg),
and no one knew who got which – neither the doctors nor the patients.
After two weeks, and then another two weeks later, the patients came
back to the hospital and got another endoscopy to see if the ulcers had
healed. After two weeks, about 30% of patients in each group had healed
ulcers. Two weeks later, things looked better. Two-thirds of the patients
taking the old drug Zantac had healed ulcers, and 88% of those people
taking the new drug, Prevacid, were better.

This is a classic example of the epitome of modern clinical medical research, what people routinely call the "gold standard" of medicine, the Randomized Controlled Trial (RCT); it is a way to provide highly objective and valuable information about what drugs work, and which ones work better than others.

Dr. Lanza and his colleagues wrote a (rather dense) scholarly article about their experiment and published it in one of the world's leading journals in this field, *The American Journal of Gastroenterology* (Lanza *et al.* 1994). There is quite a bit of discussion in the article about how the new drug might work and why it might heal up the ulcers (it has to do with restricting the amount of acid in the stomach, which seems to help create an environment where the ulcers can heal more easily). Their explanation seems plausible, and it may even account for why Prevacid works somewhat better than Zantac does.

But this experiment had another study group. Forty-four patients in the study did not receive either Zantac or Prevacid. They received what is called a "placebo," a pill which looked exactly like those the other patients took, but had no medicine in it at all; they took an "inert" pill. They had the same diagnosis, and were examined after two weeks, and again after two more weeks. And, like the other groups, no one knew which patients were taking the inert pills. What happened to them? After two weeks, about a third of the placebo patients were healed. After four weeks, just under half of them (nineteen of forty-four) were healed.

There's no discussion in Dr. Lanza's article about why *this* may have happened. What *did* happen to these people?

Whatever it was, it is very common. People have been aware for centuries that sick people, given a substance known to be inert by a doctor, frequently get better. This has, for good or ill, long been labeled the "placebo effect."

Placebo Domino: "I shall please the Lord"

The word "placebo" has a long and colorful history. In the early years of Christianity, communities of monks organized their lives with asceticism and discipline. In many communities, they developed regimens of set times for prayer and bible reading, often from the Psalms, throughout the day and night. A supplement to Vespers (often celebrated around 4:00 pm) was read and prayed when a member of the community had died. This "Office for the Dead" began with a reading of the ninth verse of Psalm 116, which, in the Latin Vulgate, says "Placebo Domino in regione vivorum," roughly translated as "I shall be pleasing to the Lord in the land of the living." "Placebo" is, in this context, usually translated as "I shall please."

Curiously, this is probably based on an inaccurate translation! The original Hebrew text has the word "eth-hal-lech" which means "I shall walk." (Note that "I shall walk with the Lord in the land of the living" makes a lot more sense than "I shall be pleasing to Him there.") When this was translated into Greek (probably sometime in the second century BCE), someone made a mistake and wrote "euarestaso", which means "I shall please." When St. Jerome translated the Bible into Latin about 500 years later, he, working from the Greek text, used the Latin word "placebo," meaning "I shall please" (Lasagna 1986).

Regardless of its origins, the term took on the somewhat different meaning in medieval English of a flatterer, sycophant, or parasite, someone out to please others with artifice rather than substance. In Chaucer's *Canterbury Tales*, written in the late fourteenth century, Chaucer tells the story of an old (two-faced) lecher named January who wants to marry a young girl; he discusses this plan with a man named Placebo, who advises him that whatever he wants to do is fine and wise, and who is he to tell January otherwise? By the early nineteenth century, this sense of the word had been adopted by physicians – a medical dictionary published in 1811 defined placebo as "an epithet given to any medicine adapted more to please than benefit the patient." One needn't know too much about the violence of medicine in 1811 – with its drastic purging and bleeding of patients (it is generally agreed by historians that George Washington was bled to death by his physicians in 1799) – to see that medical benefits were, at the time, not thought to come from anything that the patient might appreciate! And by the mid-nineteenth century it was common for people to refer to such treatments not only as "placebos" but as "*mere* placebos" – "just a divertissement to cheer the spirits, and assist the effect of the waters." By then, *water* was seen as a more effective medicine than a placebo.

In the twentieth century, as a result of the biological revolution which shook medicine to its roots, the term took on another meaning. Earlier, a placebo had been an inert substance given deliberately to please the patient (typically when the doctor didn't know what else to do). By the mid-twentieth century, it had taken on another, more complex meaning as people began to consider what was called a "second sort of placebo, the type which the doctor fancies to be an effective medicament but which later investigation proves to have been all along inert" (Houston 1938:1417–8). These drugs had been (perhaps for centuries) prescribed not to please patients, but to please doctors. And, of course, even though they were equally inert, they worked just as well as (or maybe better than) those physicians prescribed knowing them to be inert.

So, for centuries in the Western world, physicians have been aware of the fact that sick people get better after taking inert drugs. And, it should be clear that they were then (and are now) somewhat ambivalent about this. Although the reasons are complex, it must seem odd to a person who has spent twenty years learning to be a physician, studying the hundreds of medications available, to find that patients get better just because they have been in a doctor's office for a few minutes.

Why sick people get well

There are, of course, many reasons why someone might get well after getting sick. Certainly, modern pharmaceutical drugs often help the sick get better, experience less pain, heal more quickly from a variety of conditions, and, if they don't actually help heal diseases (like cold "remedies"), they often make such unhappy experiences more comfortable.

But other things happen as well. For ordinarily healthy people, most sicknesses are "self-limiting," which is a fancy way of saying that they go away by themselves. Colds and headaches are the examples with which we are most familiar. Many of the upsets of babies and small children are self-limiting; this is the origin of what must be the most common "prescription" of the pediatrician – "Call me again in the morning" – by which time the problem is usually gone. And it has long been said that, left to itself, a cold will last about a week and a half, but when treated with all the armamentarium of modern medicine will last only about ten days.

A more complicated version of this goes by the unpleasant name "regression to the mean." The idea here is that chronic diseases (ones that don't ordinarily go away "by themselves") regularly wax and wane. Such conditions get worse for a while, then get better for a while, and then worse again. And, the argument goes (although I don't think I have ever seen anyone really prove it), people tend to seek medical care when their conditions are severe. The disease is likely to start getting better by itself (at least for a while) just as the patient shows up in the doctor's office.[1] While I don't think this happens often, there clearly are situations where regression is a real factor. If people are selected for a study based on their displaying an extreme condition – like very high blood pressure, or very high levels of cholesterol – there is good reason to believe that, after some period of time, their extreme measurement will be less extreme simply because the body seeks homeostasis.

Can these factors – the self-limiting character of many illnesses and "regression to the mean" – account for the placebo effect? Certainly not.

---

[1] Consider an alternate hypothesis for which there is probably just about as much data (that is, none). The patient tends to call his doctor for an appointment at the time when his condition is worst; under managed care, he will get an appointment in about six weeks, by which time he will probably be much better.

They do account for some portion of *any* set of healing rates, although we will see that there is a good deal more to it than this.

But not without a great deal of objection. There is much objection among physicians to the very existence of something called the placebo effect. It often seems to bother doctors enormously that the *fact* of receiving medical treatment (rather than the *content* of medical treatment) can initiate a healing process. Why? I think it is because medicine is rich in a particular kind of science. Medical education is filled with science. In the US, all students must score high on the "Medical College Admission Test" in order to be admitted to medical school. Students are allowed a total of 345 minutes to complete the exam. Eighty-five minutes are devoted to "verbal reasoning," and 60 minutes to a "writing sample." The remaining 200 minutes (58%) are split evenly between "physical sciences" and "biological sciences." It is apparently important that physicians understand levers, inclined planes, the acceleration of falling bodies, the life cycle of insects, and the process of photosynthesis. The kind of science that doctors have to learn is the simpler sort of science, the mechanical kind. Physicists worked out the mechanics of simple machines (levers, planes) in the seventeenth century. In our times, they have been working on much slipperier subjects: quarks, chaos, the "weak force," and the oddest of quantum phenomena. Cause and effect are far less easy to detect in these matters than in the study of falling bodies (although "gravity" is the most complex and least understood force in physics). But it is the latter, not the former, in which physicians are schooled. And there is very little social science in medical education where one must address the complexities and subtleties of, say, emotion, or ritual, or culture. And even in the biological sciences, while there is a good deal of biochemistry, there is very little ecology, where one must try to understand cycles of relationship between predators, prey, plants, insects, and climate (for starters).

Some definitions

An education like this is extremely helpful for understanding causal relationships, where one thing causes one other thing (or seems to) – where an antibiotic kills bacteria, or physical pressure stops bleeding. But when matters get more subtle, where a drug works twice as well in one country as it does in another; where the patient gets better even though it turns out that the drug was inert; where the drug works better when it is blue than when it is red – in these kinds of cases such an education may be as much of a hindrance as a help.

Such an education can even be seen as the source of one of the very first serious obstacles to understanding these processes. Arthur K. Shapiro, MD, spent much of his career as a psychiatrist studying the placebo effect. In 1964, he proposed a definition of the placebo and the placebo effect which I will quote at length:

A placebo is defined as any therapeutic procedure (or a component of any therapeutic procedure) which is given (1) deliberately to have an effect, or (2) unknowingly and has an effect on a symptom, syndrome, disease, or patient but which is objectively without specific activity for the condition being treated. The placebo is also used as an adequate control in research. The placebo effect is defined as the changes produced by placebos. (Shapiro 1964:136)

Thirty-three years later, in a posthumously published book, Shapiro used very nearly identical words to define these same terms (Shapiro and Shapiro 1997). But this definition, with its insistence on a simplistic sort of cause and effect, is clearly impossible. The placebo is defined as "objectively without specific activity for the condition being treated." So if we put this definition in place of the word itself in the final sentence, here's what we get: "The placebo effect is defined as the changes produced by things objectively without specific activity for the condition being treated." This makes no sense whatever. Indeed, it flies clearly in the face of the obvious. The one thing that we can be absolutely sure of here is that placebos *do not* cause the placebo effect. Placebos are inert. To be inert is to not do anything. That's what inert means. If it does something (cause changes) it isn't inert. But placebos are inert, and changes do occur.

This definition confuses coincidence with cause. Just because two things occur at the same time doesn't mean that one caused the other. When a gun is fired, there is a loud noise. It happens every time. But the loud noise does not cause the hole in the target.

I suggest a very different approach to this problem. I will define what I call the *meaning response*, which is "the psychological and physiological effects of *meaning* in the treatment of illness." When such effects are "positive" (however understood), they include most of the things that have been called the placebo effect; when such effects are "negative," they include most of what has been called the nocebo effect. Since what is positive in one situation may be negative in another, this is not a fundamental distinction.[2] The meaning response includes most of the

---

[2] When you take diphenhydramine ("Benadryl") as a decongestant, if it makes you sleepy, that's negative (it's a negative "side effect"). If you take diphenhydramine ("Sleep-Eze") as a sleeping pill, and it dries your mouth and nose, that's negative (a negative "side effect"). What's positive and negative is often a matter of context and perspective.

things that have traditionally been called the placebo effect. It also may exclude a few things (which we will consider later). More important, it includes many things that are *not* part of the placebo effect as traditionally understood; we shall see that the meaning response is attached not only to the prescription of inert medications, but to active ones as well.

To show that clearly, we must first look at the whole healing process, and see what it consists of.

2　The healing process

Human beings respond to injury in three ways. *Autonomous responses* are the most important ones in healing, and involve all those processes which the organism can invoke to regain health or equilibrium, including the various immunological and related systems. A cut finger rarely needs much more than to be rinsed in water (or licked clean), and it will heal "by itself." *Specific responses* are those of the body to the content of medical treatment – to the salicylates in willow bark tea, or to the antibiotic quality of penicillin. The direct pressure of a bandage on a cut finger might facilitate its healing. *Meaning responses* follow from the interaction with the context in which healing occurs – with the "power" of the laser in surgery, or with the red color of the pill that contains stimulating medication. Sometimes, a bandage on a cut finger works better if it has a picture of Snoopy on it. These three sorts of factors all work together to enhance the sick individual's return to health.

Pain relief with "Trivaricane" and saline solution

To illustrate this threesome, I will describe the results of some research involving pain. Now pain is a tricky thing to deal with. I can't see or measure pain; I can only listen to what you say about it. And asking you about your pain is likely to change its intensity. When you have some sort of painful injury, it is often the case that, if you distract yourself – with a good book, or a movie – the pain you are experiencing may well become less intense. But when I ask you "On a scale of 1 to 10, how painful is your sprained ankle?" you are likely to attend to it directly again, and notice that "Wow! It really hurts!" when, a minute or two before, you weren't really experiencing much pain at all. So it is tricky. But there is extensive research on pain, and a lot of placebos have alleviated a lot of pain in this world, so we will be careful, and we will go ahead with the discussion.

First, it is clear that inert substances, appropriately applied, can reduce pain. Irving Kirsch, a psychologist at the University of Connecticut, has done some ingenious experiments to learn more about pain and placebos. In one experiment, he enrolled subjects – college students – in a study. The students were told they were testing a new local anesthetic called Trivaricane which had been shown to be effective in reducing pain in preliminary studies elsewhere. The placebo was a mixture of iodine, oil of thyme, and water which produced a brownish, medicinal-smelling effect when applied topically. It was in a medicine bottle labeled "Trivaricane: Approved for research purposes only." The experimenter – who wore a white lab coat and was introduced to the students as being a "behavioral medicine researcher" – put on surgical gloves and applied the placebo to one index finger or the other. If asked, the researcher said that he wore the gloves to be sure that he wasn't overexposed to the Trivaricane. Then, after a minute or so to give the medicine time to "work," a pain stimulus was applied to each index finger. The pain was applied with a mechanical gadget with a metal bar and a weight which applied a sharp force to the finger. The students were asked to rate the pain on each finger on one of several pain rating systems; in one scale, zero represented "no pain at all," and 10 represented "pain as intense/unpleasant as one can imagine." In variations of the study, the pain was applied to one finger at a time, sometimes to the placebo-treated finger first, and sometimes to that finger second; in another variation, the pain stimulus was applied at the same time to both fingers. The students routinely reported that both the intensity and the unpleasantness of the pain were less on the finger treated with the Trivaricane (Montgomery and Kirsch 1996).

There are many such studies, although this is probably the best of them. What is less common is to find such a comparison – placebo vs. no treatment of pain – outside the laboratory, in a real medical or clinical situation. But there are a few such studies. One involves a very useful and important "model" for pain research: people having wisdom teeth removed. This is a very good group of people to study for several reasons. First, tens of thousands of people have their wisdom teeth removed every year, so they are easy to find. Second, they are almost all young, strong, healthy people – between 18 and 25 – who are going to undergo a very painful and unpleasant experience from which they will in all likelihood be fully recovered in three or four days.

In this study, twenty-four people had one or more wisdom teeth removed. They received local anesthesia before the surgery but nothing else. An hour after the surgery, the patients were given a set of tests (like those in the previous study) to rate the intensity of their pain. Then twelve patients received a placebo injection while twelve received nothing. An hour later, they were given the pain tests again. The placebo-treated patients reported a substantial decrease in pain, while the untreated patients reported a substantial increase in pain; these differences were statistically significant, which means it is extremely unlikely that this outcome was due to chance (Gracely *et al.* 1979).

Why did these things happen? Why did the Trivaricane and the inert injection reduce the pain these people experienced? Remember that the one thing we can be absolutely sure of is that the stuff in the Trivaricane and the stuff in the injection (the "placebos") had nothing to do with it. And so we are left to look at what surrounds the placebos, the understandings and ideas that people have about the drugs they are taking.

Headaches and advertising

This becomes clear in a very interesting study done some years ago in England (Braithwaite and Cooper 1981). It was a large and rather complex study of the treatment of headache in 835 women. The volunteers, who all indicated that when they got headaches they treated themselves with aspirin, were divided into 4 different groups. Each person was given a packet of tablets; there were 4 different sorts of tablets distributed. "Subjects were told that the study was on behalf of a well-known manufacturer of medicines, who was comparing the effectiveness of different brands of headache tablet currently on sale." People were to take 2 tablets when they got a headache, and then to fill out a little form after an hour, indicating, among other things, how much the pain had changed on a six-point scale: -1 meant that the pain was worse; 0 meant it was the same; 1 meant that it was better; up to 4 which meant it was completely better. The trial was completely blinded; the subjects, the experimenters, and the analysts did not know who got what kind of pill until after it was over.

Group A got placebo pills labeled "analgesic tablets." Group B got the same placebo pills, but they were labeled with the brand name of one of the most popular aspirin-based drugs in the United Kingdom which "has been widely available for many years and supported by extensive advertising." Group C got aspirin tablets labeled "analgesic tablets," which looked the same as the tablets given to group A. And Group D got aspirin labeled with the same widely-advertised brand name. Figure 2.1 shows the average responses after an hour for the people in the different groups.

Now unfortunately, this study did not contain an "untreated group," a group which took no pills at all. But we know that more often than not, headaches go away by themselves, although not usually within an hour. So, by analogy with the Trivaricane study (where the placebo stopped pain

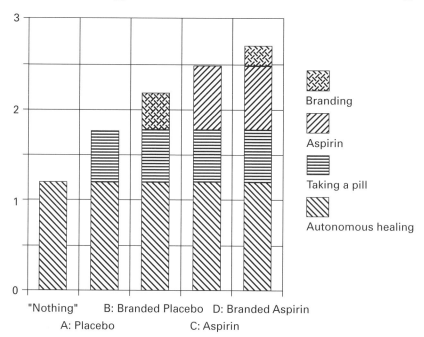

2.1 Improvement after an hour with branded or generic placebo and aspirin (*Source*: Braithwaite and Cooper 1981)

compared to "no treatment"), I have added a "no treatment" column to the outcome (labeled "Nothing"), guessing that the average amount of improvement in such a group would be small but positive. And I have carried that across the whole figure, reasoning that the headaches would be as likely to go away by themselves within an hour regardless of what medicine you might take.

So, how does it turn out? First, we can see that aspirin works better than placebo. The "Aspirin" portion of the bars (with diagonal lines) in columns C and D (aspirin and branded aspirin) can be attributed to the fact that those groups got aspirin. Now compare columns A and B (placebo and branded placebo). People who took branded placebos reported more pain relief in an hour than those who took placebos labeled "analgesic tablets." So the horizontal portion in column B has to be attributed to the fact that the placebos were labeled with a widely advertised brand name. For both groups A and B, the pills were inert; but "taking a pill" wasn't inert, and the brand name wasn't inert. Given the design of the study we can only infer the effects of taking a pill in group A, but we can be quite sure of the effect of the brand name on headache pain.

We can see the same thing in the two aspirin groups. Again, we can attribute some of the reported improvement to headaches going away by themselves (represented by diagonal bars), to the fact of taking a pill (horizontal lines), and to the fact of taking aspirin (upward diagonal bars). But we also see that the aspirin worked better with a brand name on it (crosshatching). This is a particularly important point because it indicates clearly that there is no placebo effect here. Neither group, C or D, got any placebos. D got a brand name, and it was clearly *meaningful*, just as it was for group B. Through years of advertising, these people just *knew* that this was really good aspirin. And it made a difference.

But don't forget that the aspirin helped, too. Aspirin has helped people with aches, pains, and many more serious things, for over a century; the same is true for morphine. And their natural ancestors – the salicylates found in willows, birches, wintergreen, and *Spiraea*, and opium derived from poppies – have been a comfort to people in pain for tens of thousands of years. It is largely because "pills" work at all that they work with no aspirin in them.

Conclusions

Never underestimate the ability of your body to heal herself. Human beings and other animals have rich and complex repertoires of healing processes. This is the result of tens of millions of years of evolution; natural selection favored individuals who could survive injury and overcome infection. But it is also the case that people (and some animals) have developed behavioral approaches to injury and disease; they do things to enhance healing beyond what comes as "standard equipment." People can clean wounds and splint broken bones, can provide extra nourishment for their sick children or friends, and they have an enormous experience with medicines – particularly medicinal plants – which probably reaches back 60,000 years to the middle Paleolithic (Moerman 1998b). Many of these highly effective treatments augment or enhance autonomous healing processes.

It is also apparent, however, in the cases we have seen in this chapter, that what people know and understand about medicine, what they experience about healing, what healing processes *mean* can also enhance both autonomous and behavioral healing processes. Meaning can make your immune system work better, and it can make your aspirin work better, too.

These processes – autonomous responses, as things heal by themselves; specific responses, as things are helped to heal by the application of efficacious therapies (like aspirin), and meaningful responses (like taking pills, and by brand names) – all work together to help us through illness.

Whatever else this means, it is evident that healing processes are complicated ones. Many things are going on at the same time, most of them invisible. The next chapter addresses the problem of how we can sort out these different dimensions, how we can determine what they are, and how much each contributes to the healing process.

ırement and its ambiguities

Blessing Way and Placebo Way

One of the most complex medical systems which people have developed is that of the Navajo in the four-corners region of the American Southwest. It is very common for human religious systems to revolve around elaborately ritualized meals where food is shared; the most obvious example for most readers of this book will be the Catholic mass, or similar communion ceremonies of other Christian groups, or the Passover Seder. Such shared meals are the center of ceremony in many other cultures and religions as well. The Navajo are an exception to this generalization. They do not have a meal at the center of their most significant religious rituals, but rather what we might call a visit to the doctor's office. The core of their religious life is a healing rite known as a "chant way." There are many different ceremonies used for different purposes: among them are Wind Way, Female Shooting Holy Way, Hand Trembling Evil Way, and, probably the most frequently carried out, Blessing Way. I have never found a short description of these Navajo ceremonials which seemed to describe them accurately.[3]

A typical chant way comes in several versions; it might last for two nights, five nights, or nine nights. The ceremony includes a rich complex of medicinal plants (as many as a hundred or more may be used in several different mixtures for a variety of purposes), prayers of consecration, offerings, baths, sweat baths, sandpaintings, singing all night, and so on. To oversimplify dramatically, the purpose of the event is to restore beauty or, in Navajo, *hózhó*. A person who is ill, or unhappy, or unlucky, is understood to have lost her sense of beauty, her integration with the universe. The ceremony revolves around the collection of a large set of very specific, but all very beautiful, things – plants, songs, paintings – which

---

[3] For a general account of Navajo religious healing practices see Kluckhohn and Wyman (1940); for a detailed account of Blessing Way, see Wyman (1970). For a rich account of the complexity of modern Navajo ritual healing, see Csordas (2000). A good way to gain some insight into such healing processes might be to read Leslie Marmon Silko's moving and powerful novel *Ceremony* (Silko 1988).

might be said to be focused on the *biki nahaλá*, the "patient" (Kluckhohn and Wyman 1940:13–14).

In the previous chapter, I rather blithely suggested that there were three dimensions to the healing process – autonomous, specific, and meaningful ones – and described an experiment on brand names which seemed to untangle these dimensions. But how could we possibly untangle a Blessing Way ceremony? What inert ceremony would we compare it to? What would a Placebo Way ceremony look like?

It is perfectly clear that such a complex activity, with medicinal plants, meaningful songs, chants, and sandpaintings, combined with a complex social activity, will have a broad range of meaningful and other healing elements.

One of the distinct advantages of Western medicine (at least from an analytic point of view) is that it is usually much simpler than a Blessing Way. And so it is easier to sort out these elements. But it's still not simple.

Measuring blood pressure

Many elements may be involved in a sick person getting better, and it's not always clear what they are. Consider an elaborate Australian study of the treatment of moderate hypertension: tens of thousands of Australians were screened for high blood pressure. Only those with systolic blood pressure (SBP) greater than 200 or diastolic blood pressure (DBP) greater than 90 millimeters of mercury (mm Hg) were entered in the study. Various drugs or placebos were given to different sub-groups, and the blood pressure in the participants generally dropped, as shown in measurements made every four months. The study wisely included a relatively small group of 237 untreated people with moderate hypertension – people who received no medication and no placebos of any kind – whose blood pressure was also measured every four months. Their blood pressure dropped, too. The mean DBP in this group dropped from 101.5 mm Hg (mildly elevated) to about 80 mm Hg (normal) in thirty-two months, and then stabilized at that level (plus or minus 1 mm Hg) for the next two years (MCATT 1982).

Why did the blood pressure of these people go down? For those treated with various blood pressure reducing drugs, we might be tempted to explain the decline as a result of the specific medical effectiveness of these drugs. But patients who got placebos also showed blood pressure declines. And, most interesting of all, patients who got no placebos and no medications *also* showed this decline. One explanation for the return of blood pressure to normal in this group is "regression to the mean," which we discussed briefly earlier. This principle states that, if you select a group of people based on the fact that they share an extreme characteristic (high blood pressure, for example), they will in time revert to a more normal condition as the result of ordinary human homoeostatic processes. Similarly, one can show that tall men tend to have tall sons, but not sons as tall as they are; and short men tend to have short sons, but not as short as they are. Stature tends to "regress to the mean." Note that if this were all that were going on, in some number of generations, there would no longer be any tall, or short, men. That's clearly nonsense, since it is also possible for men of average stature to have sons appreciably taller, or shorter, than they are. And that may be analogous to what happened to the people in the blood pressure study.

There are, however, other explanations. It may be that these individuals were, when first enrolled in the study, responding nervously to having their blood pressure taken, which gave them higher blood pressure; "white coat hypertension" is a well-recognized phenomenon (Landray and Lip 1999; O'Brien 1999). Having their blood pressure taken every four months may have gradually desensitized them to this event, and their blood pressure then no longer increased with the approach of the cuff. This would be a case of a distinct "measurement effect," where the measurement created the object of study, the elevated blood pressure, at least for a while.

There is another possibility: this may be an example of the meaning response. There is ample evidence to indicate that the use of various medical instruments and machines can have significant healing effects. We will look more closely at this possibility later. For the moment, we can imagine a modification to the study as I have described it which might let us make a more informed judgment about what was going on here. Suppose that the experimenters had included another group of people with high blood pressure, but the people in this group did not have their blood pressure taken every four months. Instead, their blood pressure was taken only at the end of the study, after three years. It's unlikely that this group would have gotten used to the blood pressure experience as the repeat-measurement group might have. So, if at the end of three years we found that this ignored (no treatment at all!) group *also* now had normal blood pressure, we could probably attribute the change to "regression to the mean." If that group still had high blood pressure, we could attribute the change in the multiple measurement group to the placebo effect of the blood pressure cuff. Unfortunately, the researchers didn't do this, and so we will probably never know.

The point is that it is very difficult to know, even under the most stringent conditions, and in the simplest and most clear cut cases (utterly unlike the Navajo Blessing Way), just why a particular group of people "got better." Autonomous (or homoeostatic) responses, drug responses, and meaningful responses are much easier to keep separated conceptually than they are in practice.

Diagnosis is treatment

Let's pursue this thought experiment – our addition to the Australian blood pressure study – a little bit further. Suppose we were going to do as I suggested and identified several hundred people with moderate hypertension, and then did nothing to them for three years. What might we tell them about this experiment? Unless we could measure their blood pressure without them knowing it, we would have to tell them *something*. And, we have found that their blood pressure is higher than normal. Suppose we tell a little lie; we say that they are fine, there is nothing to worry about, nothing to be done, go home and don't think about it any more. Earlier, I said that this was to be a group that got *no treatment at all*. But our little lie here doesn't seem to me to be "no treatment at all." Consider another possibility: suppose we told these people the "truth," that they had high blood pressure, that this was a risk factor for stroke and heart attack, and that they had a medical condition for which several thousand other people in this study would be treated with powerful medications. But they wouldn't get any. Of course it's unlikely that we would do either of these things; and indeed, the researchers didn't do either. But it seems quite plausible to me that if we did one or the other of these things, the outcome might have been quite different. The group to which we told lies might have been quite comforted by our charade and, as a result, their blood pressure might have gone down. The group with which we were brutally frank, but not very caring, might be expected to be scared and disturbed, and we might imagine that their blood pressure could go up, or at least not go down as it might in the group to which we lied.

What this means is that the very fact of diagnosing a person with some sort of medical condition *is a form of medical treatment* which can be expected to have an effect. This process was noticed many years ago by Howard Brody and David Waters and described in a fascinating article titled "Diagnosis is Treatment." They describe several interesting cases where it is quite clear that the shaping of the diagnosis can make a significant difference in the outcome of the illness. In one case, a 52-year-old man with long-term hypertension and recent symptoms of ulcers was quite testy with his doctor when asked about changes in his family situation. The doctor was trying to find areas of increased stress and anxiety; the patient was unwilling to describe any. But, with some persistence, the doctor learned that the man's wife had recently returned to work and was enjoying her "new life"; the patient, however, explained that he was feeling abandoned, and was very unhappy about it. The doctor suggested he discuss this with his wife. "The physician asks if he had felt more tense or sad since she returned to work. The man considers the idea and says he could not say but would think about it. He returns two weeks later to say he had discussed the conversation with his wife, who had not realized how deserted he was feeling. He is feeling much closer to her and more relaxed. He also reports a decrease in gastric pain." The authors continue by saying that in this (and another) case, "the diagnosis *in itself* exercised a therapeutic effect for the patient inasmuch as it provided an understandable, acceptable explanation for his behavior" (Brody and Waters 1980).

Untreated control groups

This leads us to another curious and complex issue. Occasionally, studies are designed to have a "no-treatment group," sometimes called a "natural history group," as did the Australian blood pressure study. The idea is that, in this group which is getting no treatment, we can see the "natural course of the disease." I would counter that, except under the most extraordinary circumstances, it is logically and conceptually impossible to have a no-treatment group. In order to do a trial, people have to be recruited and diagnosed for the condition under study; they receive some sort of examination, maybe an invasive and dramatic one. They give informed consent, perhaps after reading a long and complex document describing the study, the various treatments under review, and so on. They are then randomly assigned to (in this case) three conditions: drug treatment, placebo treatment, or no treatment. It's not clear what one will tell the group getting "no treatment." Certainly, their participation can't be "blind" to them; they know they aren't getting any drugs or placebos; a reasonable inference might be that they are healthy enough not to need any. And there has to be a follow up, an assessment of the condition of the subjects after some period of time, or a diary of symptoms has to be kept, or something similar. While these people have not had pills, they have had a good deal more than "nothing."

The only way to proceed would be to diagnose illness surreptitiously, secretly, so that the individuals didn't know they were being observed; the follow-up would also have to be secret. No lab tests would be possible. Think "medicine by binocular."

I know of only one experiment which approximates a genuine no treatment group, the Tuskegee Syphilis Study, in which the US Public Health

Service enrolled 399 poor, rural, African-American men with syphilis into a forty-year-long observational study (Jones and Tuskegee Institute 1981). The idea was, in part, to see what happened to people who had syphilis which was not treated at all. Begun in 1932, the study went on until 1972; these men were deprived of all treatment. There were moderately effective treatments with salvarsan and other drugs in the 1930s. Treatment with penicillin, which was available for treatment of syphilis in the mid-1940s, was also denied to them. In 1997, President Clinton apologized to the few survivors of the experiment and their families, and to the nation, for this egregious ethical and moral catastrophe. It is, then, *possible* to have an untreated group, but only if you are prepared to go to incredibly extreme lengths.

Clinical trials

Given this complexity, how does one ever figure anything out about medical treatment? One of the great benefits of science is that the essential methodology is simply to forge ahead anyway, regardless of the complexities, by simplifying (this, of course, is also one of the great problems of science!). The main procedure that researchers use in clinical research[4] is the "randomized controlled trial" or "RCT." An RCT is designed to determine the efficacy of a drug for people with a particular medical condition. A simple study design would go like this.

Researchers first accumulate a number of people with a certain condition. If they have lots of patients with this condition coming to their own clinic, they might just ask their own patients if they were interested in participating in the study. Or they might ask other physicians to refer appropriate patients to them. They might advertise (residents of communities with university medical centers are accustomed to seeing ads in the local newspaper saying things like "Are you a man between 25 and 40 years of age and suffering hair loss [or psoriasis, or migraine headache, or any of hundreds of other such conditions]? Call 1-888-234-5678 to participate in a study of . . . "). Recently, large research organizations like the various Institutes of the National Institutes of Health and others have been seeking participants for studies over the World Wide Web.[5] Today, many large trials are carried out simultaneously at a number of sites, from two or three to a hundred or more. Whenever such studies have any

---

[4] There is a longstanding distinction in conventional medicine between two types of research: *laboratory research* is work on chemistry or biology which might involve testing various substances on tissues grown in petrie dishes, or on animals, and perhaps on the occasional "human guinea pig," or the like. *Clinical research* involves testing drugs or procedures on human beings in hospitals, doctors' offices, or clinics.

[5] For example, see http://cancertrials.nci.nih.gov/ for the NIH "cancerTrials" page.

federal funding, and most other times, too, they have been approved by a research committee – often called an Institutional Review Board (IRB) – to see that they are ethically acceptable, that the rights of the patients who volunteer for the trials are protected, and, particularly, to see that all patients are appropriately asked for their "informed consent."

Patients are then matched up against the entrance requirements for the study. This is a very important point in the process. Sometimes, it's relatively simple: "patients with active ulceration of the duodenum as seen on endoscopy" is pretty straightforward; "patients with significant late-luteal phase dysphoric disorder (i.e., PMS)," or, remembering our earlier discussion, "patients with mild to moderate hypertension" are more problematic. Let's take the simpler case: ulcers.

After being selected for the study, patients are given some sort of treatment for the condition. In some studies, there will be three or four treatment groups with different amounts of medication (10 mg, 20 mg, 30 mg, etc.). In the technical argot of medicine, these are sometimes called "verum" groups; verum means "true" or "truly." And then there is also a "control group." The control group may be given an existing standard drug or it may be given an inert treatment, a "placebo." The central necessities at this stage are that patients must be allocated to the different treatment groups *at random*, and that neither the researchers nor the patients can know who is getting which treatment; hence they are called "Randomized Controlled Trials."

The patients are treated with their medications or placebos for an appropriate length of time – in the case of ulcers, it might be for about a month – and then they are checked again to see what has happened; they might receive a second endoscopic examination, for example. At this point, the study is "unblinded," and the outcome in the treatment groups is compared. For the sake of simplicity, let's assume that there were two groups, one receiving active drug treatment and one receiving placebo treatment. And suppose we find that, in the drug treatment group, 60% of the patients are better, while in the placebo treatment group, 40% are better. Sounds pretty good.

But suppose that we had only 10 people in each group. In the drug group, 6 of 10 were better, while in the placebo group, 4 of 10 were better. There are only 2 more in the drug group that got better than in the placebo group. It seems pretty likely that this could have occurred simply by chance; we might very well have had this outcome if we had given placebos (or active drugs) to both groups. Indeed, this example is rather like the outcome of an experiment of flipping coins. Flip a coin 10 times, and you have an excellent chance of getting 6 heads one time, and 4 the next. If, however, you flip the same coin 1,000 times, it is extremely unlikely that you will get 600 heads the first time round and 400 heads the second. If you had a crooked coin, you might get heads 606 once and 594 once, but not 600 and then 400. So, sample size is important.

Suppose in our ulcer treatment study we had enrolled 2,000 patients, and we had 60% healed in the drug group (600 of 1000), and 40% in the placebo group (400 of 1,000). It seems extremely likely that, if we repeated this experiment, we would *not* get reversed results the second time, just like the coin. It is quite clear that we can conclude now that the drug is an effective one for healing ulcer disease. But we have had to do an *awful* lot of work to prove it, studying 2,000 patients. This is why the use of statistics is essential in doing clinical research. Using fairly straight-forward statistics, one can determine what the probability is that the out-come of a particular experiment is due to chance. For example, when you flip a coin 10 times, you have a 37% probability of getting 6 heads; such an outcome is likely 1 time in 3. No one is likely to conclude from this experiment that we have a biased coin (or an effective drug).

If, however, we have 50 patients in each of two groups, one getting an active drug and one getting a placebo, and 60% of the drug patients are better (30 of 50) at the end of the trial, and 40% of the placebo patients are better (20 of 50), there is only a 4.5% chance that this "biasing" of the outcome is due to chance. In such a case, it is common to say that there is less than one chance in 20 (5%) that the outcome is due to chance; people also say that the result is "statistically significant at the .05 level."

Now notice that just because something is "statistically significant" doesn't necessarily mean that it is particularly important (or "signifi-cant"). If we have a new drug that we test on 10,000 people (two groups of 5,000 each), and people in the drug group are better at the end of the trial 51% of the time (2550 of 5,000), and the placebo group patients are better 49% of the time (2,450 of 5,000), this is a statistically signifi-cant difference which is exactly the same as in the previous case (this outcome could happen simply due to chance only 4.5% of the time). But even though the difference is statistically significant, it doesn't seem very significant (unless it were really really cheap to do!).

Another way to look at this is to use the concept of the Number Needed to Treat (NNT). The NNT tells you how many people have to receive some treatment in order for one person to benefit from it. To calculate the NNT, you determine the proportion of benefit the treatment gives, and divide it into 100. In our case with 50 patients in each group, where 60% of drug patients got better, and 40% of control patients got better, the proportion of benefit is 60% – 40% which equals 20%, which we divide into 100% giving an NNT of 5. We need to treat 5 patients with the new drug in order for one to benefit. All 5 have to pay for the drug, and all 5 have to tolerate its undesirable effects, and one will benefit. In our case with 10,000 patients, the proportion of benefit is 51% – 49%, or 2%, which divided into 100% gives an NNT of 50. We have to treat 50 people with this new drug to have one person benefit. Just because a difference is "statistically significant" doesn't mean it is "significant" for real medical practice.

Note that I have been assuming that the differences between the drug group and the control group in these studies was due to the fact that one group got the drug and the other didn't. Are there any other possibilities? One of the biggest problems in doing RCTs is being certain that the individuals were assigned to the different groups in a truly random fashion. Suppose, for example, that the researchers decided to simplify, and arranged for all the men to be in one group and all the women to be in the other. This would hardly be a random distribution. Indeed, it is common enough for researchers to restrict study subjects to one gender or the other (it has traditionally been men) just so this couldn't arise. At the end of the study, when the results are "unblinded," the researchers compare the two groups on a variety of demographic measures, hoping that there are no differences – in gender, age, illness severity, economic status, etc. – between them. If the groups are the same on these measures, it is taken as evidence that the two groups are "the same," and therefore any differences between them are due to the presence or absence of the drug being tested.[6]

There is another factor to consider. It is often alleged that, for a variety of reasons, RCTs aren't really "blind." In particular, it is said that people can figure out who is taking the drug and who is taking the placebo by noticing "side effects," or whatever. This may be the case. In so far as it is, and in so far as doctors or researchers convince people who researchers think to be taking the drug that they will do better than others, the results of the trial will probably show a deflated "placebo effectiveness" rate and an inflated "verum effectiveness" rate. Later, if the drug is approved for use, practicing physicians, convinced by these biased studies that the drug is highly effective, will convey that enthusiasm (or bias) to their patients and may heal a lot of patients with the meaning response. There's nothing

---

[6] There is a down side to this. If you pick your patients so they are all white men between 40 and 45 with "stage II illness," who each make between $37,000 and $40,000 per year in middle management, and don't wear glasses, and then randomly assign them to different groups, at the end you will be able to show that the two groups were "the same." But you won't have any real idea of whether your new drug will be of any value for rich 20-year-old black women, or 70-year-old nearsighted Hispanics. This is a very common problem in medicine; in particular, most drugs have, over the years, not been tested in women or children.

wrong with this, of course, but it's likely that, if some skeptic comes along later with a better research design and tests the drug again, it will disappear from the pharmacies fairly quickly.

The very fact that conventional medicine relies so strongly on the randomized controlled trial, often referred to as the "gold standard" of medicine, rests on the fact that people get better when they take inert medications. We now turn to a consideration of why and how this happens.

4   Doctors and patients

The standard explanation for why people respond to placebos is a psychological one: people are suggestible, or they are neurotic, or something like that. But consider an interesting experiment described by Richard Gracely, one of the leading pain researchers in the United States. It shows clearly that clinicians – doctors, dentists, nurses, and so on – play a very important role in this response.

What the doctor knows makes a difference

Sixty people who were having their wisdom teeth removed participated in an experiment designed by Dr. Gracely. They were told they would receive either placebo (which might reduce the pain of having the tooth removed, or might do nothing), naloxone (which might increase their pain, or do nothing), fentanyl (which might reduce their pain, or do nothing), or no treatment at all. Subjects were all recruited from the same patient stream, with consistent selection criteria by the same staff. The tricky part of the experiment is this: What Gracely was actually studying was not so much patients as *clinicians.* In the first phase of the study, the clinicians (the dentists and nurses) – but not the patients – were told fentanyl was not yet a possibility because of administrative problems with the study protocol, yielding the PN group. In the second phase, a week later, clinicians were told that the problems had been resolved, and now patients might indeed receive fentanyl, yielding the PNF group. Figure 4.1 shows the effects of placebo treatment in the two groups. "Pain after placebo administration in group PNF was significantly less than pain after placebo in group PN at 60 minutes (t[23df] = 3.56, p < .01). The two placebo groups differed only in the clinician's knowledge of the range of possible double-blind treatments" (Gracely *et al.* 1985). Note that Dr. Gracely attributed this difference not to the varying personalities of the dentists involved, but to their knowledge. And somehow, without even realizing it, these clinicians conveyed to their patients (who were receiving inert medication) that they *might* receive a powerful painkiller

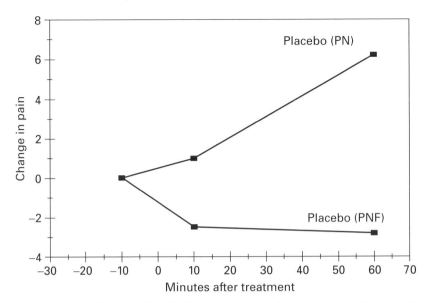

4.1   Effects of physician knowledge on patient response to inert medication (*Source*: Gracely *et al.* 1985)

(PNF group) or they might *not* (PN group). And this was sufficient to make a substantial and statistically significant difference in the experience of their patients, to soothe the pain of the extraction of wisdom teeth; remember that the patients represented in the figure are only those who received placebo injections. These two patient groups are similar to the two placebo groups in the study we looked at in Chapter 2 on brand name aspirin; except this time, the "reputation" of the inert treatment came not from a brand name, but from physician knowledge and enthusiasm.

Patient psychology and the search for "placebo responders"

The traditional approach to this issue has been quite different, and has focused on the psychological characteristics of patients. The standard experimental design was to divide a group of patients or experimental subjects into two groups, a group which responded to a placebo of some sort and a group which didn't. These groups were then compared on a variety of personality measures. These studies have yielded a variety of results indicating, for example, that placebo responders were more neurotic and extroverted than nonreactors in one study (Gartner 1961), more "acquiescent" in another (Fisher and Fisher 1963), "outgoing, verbally and socially skilled, and generally well adjusted" as opposed to "belligerent, aggressive and antagonistic to authority" in another (Muller 1965), tending to exhibit "higher anxiety and lower ego strength and self-sufficiency" in another (Walike and Meyer 1966), and so on. So, placebo reactors are neurotic yet well-adjusted, outgoing and socially skilled yet acquiescent to authority, extroverted yet with low ego strength. No one has ever been able to find a reliable way to predict who is going to respond to inert treatment and who is not (Liberman 1967; Fisher 1967).

It is also important to note that the same people respond differently at different times to medication, active or inert; the response is very inconsistent. In a classic study in the 1950s, researchers – working with Veteran's Hospital inpatients with sleep disturbances – studied the possible uses of an antihistamine (methapyrilene hydrochloride) as a hypnotic to induce sleep. They tell us that "No patient was accepted for the study who . . . was a known placebo reactor". They aren't clear on just how they knew this, but they tried. They then gave varying drugs – active or inert – to their subjects to see their influence on sleep. "Although all known placebo reactors were excluded from the study, it was found that over 30% of the patients scored the placebo as excellent in inducing and maintaining sleep" (Straus, Eisenberg, and Gennis 1955).

Similarly, many contemporary studies, especially of chronic conditions, begin with some sort of "placebo washout" or "run-in" stage; in these cases, patients are given inert medication for several weeks before the study actually begins (Knipschild, Leffers, and Feinstein 1991; Lang 1992; Knipschild, Leffers, and Feinstein 1992). Researchers are rarely very clear about why they are doing this, but there seem to be two reasons: one more overt, one more covert. The overt reason is to "clear the patient of any previous medication," while the more covert is to eliminate what Straus and his colleagues in the 1950s called "known placebo responders." This technique is common in studies of hypertension. In such studies, patients with blood pressure over a certain level are entered into the trial, then given inert medication for three to five weeks; individuals whose blood pressure falls below the low-level cutoff point for entry into the study are then usually dropped from the trial. Such studies have a bias against individuals responsive to meaningful treatment. These "washout/run-in" rates can be substantial. In one study from Hong Kong, 16 of 52 patients (31%) originally recruited were excluded because their blood pressure dropped below entry requirements for the study after four weeks of placebo treatment (Chan *et al.* 1992). In a study in the United States, 125 of 507 recruited patients (25%) were dropped during the four-to-six week placebo lead-in phase, "most often because their diastolic blood pressure fell below 92 mmHg" (Schoenberger and

Wilson 1986:381). In the Chinese trial, even after eliminating a third of the patients for responding to placebos, the mean diastolic blood pressure (mDBP) of the control group patients dropped from 104 to 97, while the mDBP of the drug group (taking nebivolol) dropped from 99 to 83. In the American study, even after eliminating a quarter of the patients, the mDBP of the control group dropped from 98 to 95 while the drug treatment group (taking captopril) mDBP dropped from 100 to 92. One cannot eliminate "placebo responders" from a trial.

This has also been shown in a large study of drug trials for the treatment of depression: "Metaanalyses[7] of 101 studies reveal that a placebo run-in does not (1) lower the placebo response rate, (2) increase the drug-placebo difference, or (3) affect the drug response rate" after the patients are randomized to drug and placebo treatment (Trivedi and Rush 1994).

So, you can't identify in advance those people who might respond to inert medication. And if you try to do so using, for example, a placebo run-in, it won't make any difference in the outcome (except that you will have a smaller sample size). The general conclusion is that the characteristics and qualities of individual patients make no significant impact on the character and quality of meaning effects. What then does make a difference?

Doctor effects and the search for "placebogenesis"

It seems quite clear that the most important single factor shaping the meaningful quality of medicine springs from doctors. Consider the following text, the testimony of a 76-year-old veteran of the Second World War, who was one of ten men in a study of knee surgery (Moseley *et al.* 1996). Although he didn't know it for certain until somewhat later, he had been one of five in the study to have sham surgery on his knee to treat his arthritis; he was mildly anaesthetized and given three stab wounds in the knee to mimic the visible results of arthroscopic surgery. And it worked quite nicely. Here, the patient describes the outcome of his surgery, and his surgeon, Dr. Bruce Moseley:

I was very impressed with him, especially when I heard he was the team doctor with the [Houston] Rockets.... So, sure, I went ahead and signed up for this new thing he was doing ... The surgery was two years ago and the knee never has bothered me since. It's just like my other knee now. I give a whole lot of credit to Dr. Moseley. Whenever I see him on TV during a basketball game, I call the wife in and say, "Hey, there's the doctor that fixed my knee." (Talbot 2000)

---

[7] A "metaanalysis" or "meta-analysis" is a special kind of comparison of a large number of related studies which allows one to make inferences which the studies, taken one at a time, might not allow. It is, in effect, an analysis of a series of analyses.

Surely this man's knee was healed by Dr. Moseley, not by three stab wounds, but in some more complex and much more interesting way. I have met and spoken with Bruce Moseley, and I agree with the arthroscopy patient. He is a very impressive man. He's tall, strong, and athletic looking. He has a firm, friendly, and persuasive manner. I'm not certain how I "know" something like this, but he sure looks like a good surgeon to me even though I've never seen him on TV, and I'm not much of a basketball fan.

That is the general finding of most of the research looking into these matters. In 1938, W. R. Houston told the American College of Physicians, meeting in St. Louis, about "The Doctor Himself as a Therapeutic Agent." He urged the adoption of a higher scientific medicine, one which would allow the "doctor himself, as therapeutic agent, [to] be refined and polished to make of himself a more potent agent," adding that this would "lead to the physician's occupying a position of even greater dignity in the social order than the high place he now holds" (Houston 1938).

Arthur K. Shapiro, one of the most eminent students of the placebo effect, described a variation on this theme which he called "the indirect interest of the physician in the patient." He derived this perspective from a complex case of his where a depressed woman, whenever treated with any medication, immediately developed a long and intolerable list of physical complaints requiring her doctor to stop her treatment. Shapiro prescribed for her "an elaborate dosage schedule of twelve placebo tablets daily." She reacted, as in the past, with multiple physical complaints. He then told her that she had been taking inert placebos "to convince her that the symptoms were caused by psychological factors and not by the medication." Subsequently, he treated her with imipramine (Tofranil), and she got much better without the kinds of complaints she had previously experienced. He then considers what factors might have accounted for her improvement.

This patient's remarkable response was probably more related to my interest in the treatment than to any other factor. It is obvious that I am intellectually and emotionally interested in the placebo phenomenon and therefore in this patient's negative placebo response. The management was an attempt to explore and innovate a treatment procedure. There was an element of danger in my not knowing how the patient would respond; she did consider suicide for a short period following the confrontation. In other words, my interest in the phenomenon was experienced by the patient as an interest in her.

Several years later the patient told Shapiro that she had understood that he " 'was really trying to help her' . . . whereas physicians previously 'were too busy,' uninterested, and 'would only give her boxes of pills'; and that she was then 'able to have faith in the clinic and doctors' which enabled her to take medication and finally improve" (Shapiro 1964). Shapiro's perspective – that the patient's understanding (knowledge) of the physician's interest in her, genuine or not (she interpreted his interest in his experiment as interest in her) – seems to me to be as productive as it is (surprisingly) honest.

John Whitehorn did ingenious research in the 1950s with psychiatrists working with schizophrenic patients. He noticed that some doctors (whom he called "A") had substantially better results with their patients than others ("B") did; three-quarters of A doctors' patients improved while only a quarter of B doctors' did. He examined the doctors, and found that there were persistent differences in the ways they responded to questions on the Strong Vocational Interest Test. He noted "definite differences in the interest patterns [in 4 vocations] of the A and B physicians. These 4 vocations are lawyer and C.P.A. (A's high B's low); Printer and Mathematics Physical Science Teacher (A's low B's high)." In a much closer examination of these test scores, Whitehorn came to some interesting conclusions about this difference. The A's, he wrote, "resembling lawyers, [may] have a problem-solving . . . approach [while] B doctors, with attitudes resembling printers – black or white, right or wrong – are likely to view the patient as a wayward mind needing correction" (Whitehorn and Betz 1960).[8]

There is also experimental evidence which bears on this issue and can be interpreted in the same way. A pioneering and elegant study by Uhlenhuth, for example, showed that the mild tranquilizer meprobamate (Elavil) was more effective than placebo in treating anxious outpatients only in one of three clinics, and then only when physicians adopted a very positive "therapeutic" attitude through which they "maintained a solicitous, confident and enthusiastic attitude, [toward the patient, and] . . . communicated a pervasive assurance that the medication was effective for his particular complaint," etc. In the same clinic, when physicians adopted an "experimental" attitude – "detached, uncertain and observing, . . . [and] communicated to the patient that the medication was as yet of uncertain value for the patient's condition" – there was no difference in outcome between drug and placebo groups, and both groups did worse than the patients with the enthusiastic physician (Uhlenhuth *et al.* 1966).

This finding was confirmed by an even more complex study which compared four variables – the status of the communicator (dentist vs. technician), the attitude of the dentist, the attitude of the dental technician, and the message of drug effects – on the effectiveness of a placebo.

---

[8] Then again, I have a brother who's a printer. Believe me, not all printers are "black or white, right or wrong" kind of guys.

The subjects in the study were dental patients who were given a pill (an inert capsule) before they received a mandibular block injection of local anesthetic (the shot you get in the jaw before dental work). Then they were asked to rate the pain of the injection. The amount of pain varied depending on just what they were told, and who told them. The most important factor was the message of the drug effect. Patients were given either an "Oversell message" ("This is a recently developed pill that I've found to be very effective in reducing tension, anxiety, and sensitivity to pain. It cannot harm you in any way. The pill becomes effective almost immediately") or an "Undersell message" ("This is a recently developed pill that reduces tension, anxiety and sensitivity to pain in some people. Other people receive no benefit from it. I personally have not found it to be very effective. It cannot harm you in any way. The pill becomes effective almost immediately if it's going to have an effect.") Patients who received the Oversell message "exhibited the least pain from the injection and significant post-placebo reductions in both . . . anxiety and fear of injection." The message was much more significant than the "attitude" of the dentist or technician – a warm versus a neutral attitude to the patient (Gryll and Katahn 1978). In this case, the patient's knowledge (even though based on "false" information) trumped the "chair side manner" of the professionals.

In a more recent study of general practice consultation, Thomas showed the effect of a "positive" diagnosis compared with a more neutral approach on the part of the physician. A series of 200 patients with symptoms but no abnormal physical signs (characteristic of roughly half of office visits to the general practitioner) were randomly assigned to a "positive" consultation with or without a prescription (of a generally neutral drug – 3 mg tablets of thiamine hydrochloride), or a "negative" or "neutral" consultation with or without the same prescription. In the positive consultations, "the patient was given a firm diagnosis and told confidently that he would be better in a few days." In the negative consultations, the doctor said "I cannot be certain of what is the matter with you." In a survey of patients two weeks later, 64% of positive consultation patients said they were all better, while only 39% of those who had negative consultations thought they were better ($p < .001$; this could occur as a chance result less than one time in a thousand experiments). Receiving a treatment in this study made no difference; physician attitude to the patient's illness overrode any consideration of the pills patients might have received (Thomas 1987).

Herbert Benson and David McCallie reviewed the medical literature on the history of the medical treatment of angina pectoris (1979). They found that in the recent past, in the 1940s and 1950s just before the age of the double blind trial, there were a number of drugs which had been in widespread use for treating angina and which had been intensively studied. They also noted that a number of these drugs, after being in widespread use, were subjected to placebo controlled trials. In those trials, the drugs were no more effective than the placebos! They note a consistent pattern: "The initial 70 to 90 percent effectiveness in the enthusiasts' reports decreases to 30 to 40 percent 'base-line' placebo effectiveness in the [later] skeptics' reports" (Benson and McCallie 1979:1424). Thus, for this grave condition, skeptics can heal 30% to 40% of their patients with inert medication, while enthusiasts can heal 70% to 90%. There is little reason to think that, in the studies Benson reviewed, the later doctors attracted to them more skeptical patients. The difference here is that enthusiastic doctors could heal twice as many people as skeptical ones could with the same drugs.

So far we have seen that the doctors' attention (or "indirect interest," their interest in the patient as a "case"), their aptitudes (as lawyers or printers), and their attitudes and enthusiasms all make a difference; all can influence patients and can enhance (or retard) their healing processes. But how are these factors conveyed to patients? What sorts of communication have effects?

Doctor–patient communication

Moira Stewart recently reviewed a large number of studies which, in a way, bear on this problem. She wanted to know if the quality of physician–patient communication made a significant difference in patient health outcomes. She found, generally, that they did. But she focused more on the *form* of communication than on its *content*. She compared several studies involving patient choice: "In one (Morris and Royle 1988), the fact that a woman [with breast cancer] was able to choose the kind of breast surgery to have was not found to be related to emotional health outcomes. In another (Fallowfield *et al.* 1990), going to a surgeon who permitted (but did not force) the choice *was* found to be related to positive outcomes. I would suggest, therefore, that it was not simply the decision-making power of the patient that was effective but, rather, the provision of a caring, respectful and empowering context in which a woman was enabled to make an important decision with both support and comfort" (Stewart 1995:1422–3). It is also possible to put another interpretation on this. In the study cited, women were assigned to physicians of three sorts: those who preferred mastectomy; those who preferred lumpectomy; or those who offered their patients a choice of treatment. The women who saw the third type of physician had less post-operative depression

Table 4.1. *Elements of effective discussion of the medical management plan*

Element	Patient outcomes affected
Patient is encouraged to ask more questions	Anxiety (Thompson, Nanni, and Schwankovsky 1990), role limitation and physical limitation (Greenfield, Kaplan, and Ware 1985; Kaplan, Greenfield, and Ware 1989; Greenfield *et al.* 1988).
Patient is successful at obtaining information	Functional status (Greenfield, Kaplan, and Ware 1985; Kaplan, Greenfield, and Ware 1989) and physiological status (Kaplan, Greenfield, and Ware 1989; Greenfield *et al.* 1988)
Patient is provided with information programs and packages	Pain (Egbert *et al.* 1964), function (Johnson *et al.* 1988), mood and anxiety (Rainey 1985)
Physician gives clear information along with emotional support	Psychologic distress (Roter and Hall 1991), symptom resolution (Heszen-Klemens and Lapinska 1984), blood pressure (Orth *et al.* 1987)
Physician and patient agree about the nature of the problem and the need for follow-up	Problem (Starfield *et al.* 1981) and symptom (Bass *et al.* 1986) resolution
Physician is willing to share decision making	Patient anxiety (Fallowfield *et al.* 1990)

Source: Stewart 1995.

than women treated by either of the other two types. It could be that the physicians who gave women a choice had to explain the benefits and costs of both procedures, rather than only explaining one. Hence the woman with choice had more real information, she knew more, and the physician shared with her the knowledge; that is, both were in agreement on the better way to proceed. Stewart also notes that "agreement between physician and patient was found to be a key variable that influenced outcomes (Starfield *et al.* 1981; Bass *et al.* 1986)."

Table 4.1, redrawn from Stewart's article, can be similarly interpreted. In each case, one can infer that the patient actually gained some information from the physician, and probably came to understand something of the level of the physician's commitment to it (compared to some sort of relevant control); in each case, there was some evidence of symptom mitigation. In the first row of the table, for example, one study has shown that, when patients were encouraged to ask questions, anxiety was reduced; in three additional studies, such encouragement led to an improvement in role and physical limitation. Knowledge can mitigate the effects of illness.

Conclusions

What we find here is, first, that the psychological makeup or the personality of the patient has little to do with the outcome of a medical procedure, and, in particular, that one cannot predict who will respond to inert medication by referring to patient character. By contrast, there is ample evidence to indicate that the nature, character, personality, behavior, and style of doctors can influence a good deal of human response not only to inert but also to active medication. It is as if the physician's demeanor activates medication, inert or otherwise. I think it is probably the case that the most important aspect of that demeanor is its "certainty." This might appear as enthusiasm, but need not, at least not in the sense of the "enthusiastic cheerleader." A common quality of clinicians the world around, regardless of how they understand their practice, is a quiet assurance, a certainty, that things will turn out well. Hence, successful clinicians will have a deep and abiding commitment to the character and nature of their techniques.

An ethnographic anecdote: in the later 1990s, I attended a conference with a number of people interested in the placebo effect. A meeting was held to consider forming some sort of association addressing this area of interest. As is common at such meetings, everyone was asked to introduce him or herself. Near the back of the room, seated next to one another, were two Korean-American gentlemen, both of them acupuncturists. I had observed them earlier in animated and friendly conversation. However, after the first had introduced himself, and while the second was doing so, the first realized something about the acupuncture technique of the second. Unlike himself, who used a "deep needling" technique, the second used a "shallow needling" technique. Unable to contain himself, the first loudly interrupted the second's self-introduction, saying "But that means your whole technique is based on the placebo effect!!" The second shouted back to the effect that, no, it was the first practitioner's technique that was "all placebo." Although they did not come to blows, a budding friendship foundered on the shoals of the placebo effect. More important, the incident shows how deep and fundamental was the commitment of each to his own technique. Of course, a biomedically trained internist or surgeon (more polite than our acupuncturists) might have muttered to himself that the techniques of both were "only" the placebo effect. The sheer intensity of this interchange can show us something important about how any sort of healing might work, and how important the healer's commitment to the method is to its success.

In a similar way, but from another direction, it is a commonplace in the non-Western world that many people who become healers of some sort or other are those who have been cured of some serious illness by the medical system they subsequently join. Edgerton's famous account of Abedi, a "traditional African psychiatrist," is a good example. Abedi turned to a specialization in mental illnesses after suffering a series of hallucinations which occurred at the beginning of his medical apprenticeship with his father. He was terrorized when he heard voices of people he couldn't see; it was weeks later before he was cured of this bout of illness which was diagnosed as being due to witchcraft. He had a long subsequent career curing the most violently psychotic individuals (Edgerton 1971).

For a more recent case, see the marvelous account of "Sister Grace," a Navajo Catholic nun who blended charismatic Christianity, elements of both the Native American Church (NAC) and classical Navajo tradition, and conventional Western medicine in her healing ministry, which began after her immersion in these traditions led to her emergence from a profound depression. She has become a very well known and respected healer on the Navajo reservation. Sister Grace's father, healed from an accident with help from the Native American Church, himself became an accomplished "roadman" of the NAC (Begay and Maryboy 2000).

The personal experience of these people is, in itself, undeniable evidence, powerful proof for them of the power and usefulness of their healing art. This is uncommon in biomedicine – the great majority of oncologists have not had cancer; most cardiologists do not have heart disease; few geriatric specialists seem much older than forty. The only persistent exception in (or, perhaps, at the margins of) conventional medicine is for psychiatrists who specialize in psychoanalysis; it is still generally the case that psychoanalysts have undergone psychoanalysis during their training (and usually continue it during their practice). The changes which this experience brings to their lives – like those that transform the man or woman who becomes a shaman – can be powerful and convincing evidence of its effectiveness.[9]

---

[9] If there is a common thread among many autobiographical accounts of physicians who have experienced serious illness, it is their shock and dismay at how hard, how humiliating, how exhausting, and how painful it can be to be a patient; Robert Hahn has written a thoughtful and interesting review, titled "Between Two Worlds," of the ways doctors report on their experience with serious illness (Hahn 1995: 234–61). Here, for example, is some testimony from a nephrologist who, diagnosed with metastatic lung cancer, had to have chemotherapy, among other things:

I have spent a tremendous percentage of my time telling my patients that they needed to show up for dialysis, needed to stay for the full treatment. I have heard every type of excuse for cutting times and treatments. Some patients have cussed me out. One said "Get out of my face." Another said, "You have no idea what it is like to go through this." I have sometimes become unpopular among patients because I would not accept the selfish remark, "It's my life." My response, "But what about your wife, your little children and

But for more ordinary physicians, who have not experienced the treatments they prescribe for their patients, other devices must serve to create this assurance. In Western medicine, the primary device for achieving this end is the extraordinary romance medicine has with science. Medical students are steeped in science. Doctors routinely argue that their work "is scientific." By this, they mean that it is somehow based on real scientific analysis or experiment; that is, that it's "true." Modern medical education is steeped in science – from the MCATs to the fixation on "data"; "show me the data" is the first thing any doctor will ever ask. When I explained to my family doctor once that a recurring minor but annoying skin problem seemed to abate when I took a course of antibiotics for some other condition, she laughed and said, "Well, you're ahead of the data on that one!" And, of course, much of medicine *is* based on real scientific research and practice. But much of it is not. Much medicine, probably a majority of it, is based on clinical experience, on the experience of doctors in their clinical rounds. There is, for example, no scientific evidence to support giving antibiotics to children with sore throats except under the most stringent and special circumstances; a review of studies of treatment of 10,484 cases of sore throat showed that antibiotics shortened the duration of symptoms by 8 hours over the course of an illness lasting about a week or 10 days (Del Mar, Glasziou, and Spinks 2000). Yet, regardless of evidence, it is done all the time. There are many other similar examples (Moerman 1998a). But it doesn't really matter given the issue we are addressing. What is important is that doctors – healers of any sort or type – are *convinced* that their techniques are powerful and effective, and that there is undeniable evidence of this effectiveness. In some places, such proof comes from gods or spirits, in some places from personal experience, and in other places from the assertions of science. In so far as these convictions are somehow conveyed to patients and, in the process, convince *them* of their doctor's power, then they are likely (within the bounds of our physical mortality) to *be* effective.

grandchildren, your friends. It is selfish to rob them of your beauty just because you are too impatient to sit in a chair for four hours." Maybe it is fate, but my chemotherapy time is the exact time as my average patient's dialysis – four hours. I go to a state hospital, and sometimes have to wait two and a half hours to be put on. I have a pesky pump as my companion, and can either watch boring soap operas, read or sleep. I can complain, laugh, or cry. There is only one thing, and one thing only I cannot let myself do – cut my time short . . . With a great deal of humbleness and humility to my patients, I can now very safely proclaim, "It is a lot easier to be the doctor than the patient." (Fadem 2000)

For another view of this situation, watch William Hurt in *The Doctor*, where a surgeon learns what medicine is really like after he contracts cancer. This film is often shown to medical students.

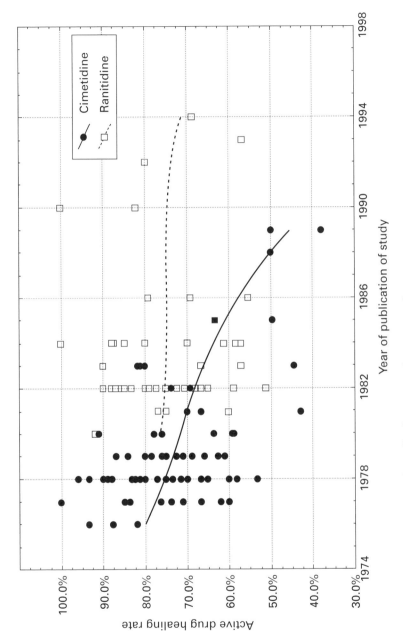

4.2 Old drugs become less effective as new drugs come along

In August, 1920, my wife's great-grandfather, her mother's father's father, wrote some memoirs of his life. Born in 1840, he had trained in Strasbourg, France to be a physician. After about twenty years of practice, he began to doubt his abilities: "My feeling of being impotent against the fatal progress of most diseases drove me little by little to be disgusted with the practice of medicine. It is obvious that a doctor, to exercise his profession properly and not become a charlatan, must be convinced that his prescriptions can only have a favorable effect on the course of the disease." Losing this conviction, Dr. Schmidt left medicine and became a tax collector.

The ways in which doctors convince themselves of the effectiveness of their techniques changes through time. For example, I cited above Dr. Houston's account of "The Doctor Himself as a Therapeutic Agent." This paper (the record of a distinguished address to the American College of Physicians in 1938) contained not a single reference, no charts, no data at all. The paper by Dr. Stewart with which I brought the discussion to a close, published in 1995, compared the results of 21 randomized controlled trials which examined the effects of various interventions in 3,753 different patients. Both papers seem quite convincing; but the styles of evidence and presentation, and the sense of what it means to be "scientific," have changed.

It is also important to note that doctors don't really have to work very hard at this much of the time. Look again at Figure 4.1 at the beginning of this chapter, and recall that the difference in pain relief these patients experienced after receiving inert medication can be attributed to the fact that, in the PNF group, the doctors, but not the patients, knew that these patients *might* get fentanyl (which is certainly very effective) and that those patients in the PN group would not get it. It's not that they got it – all the patients represented in the figure got an injection of sterile saline solution – it was that the doctors knew they *might* get it. The cues being given to patients in a situation like this are extremely subtle; indeed, no one has any idea what they are. But doctors *know* that fentanyl is potent stuff, and just the possibility of your getting it is likely to reduce your pain.

Finally, to make the case that it is doctors, not patients, who are the primary active ingredient here, one can demonstrate the proposition that old treatments become less effective as new treatments come along. Figure 4.2[10] shows the results of 117 studies of treatment of gastric ulcers with two different drugs (Moerman 2000). The points show the percentage of people in each study who were healed by the drug (based on an endoscopic examination). The studies are plotted in terms of their dates

---

[10] The graph was made using the Statistica software package, using negative exponentially-weighted fitting.

of publication. The points represented by solid circles are studies of one of the first really effective treatments for ulcer disease, cimetidine (tradename Tagamet), a drug which inhibits the production of acid in the gut. The earliest studies were done in 1975, and they continued for about ten years. But in 1981, the first studies were done of a new, "better" drug which also blocked acid called ranitidine (tradename Zantac). Before ranitidine came along in 1981, cimetidine healed 72% of the patients treated with it in trials. After ranitidine came along, the effectiveness of cimetidine dropped so that only 64% of patients treated with it were cured; ranitidine cured 75% of patients treated with it in trials. It is, of course, research physicians (those doing these studies), not patients, who are fully aware of (and excited by) newly emerging drugs. As they convey their enthusiasm for their new drugs, they may simultaneously disparage the "older" ones, even though they may not be aware they are doing it.

In summary, what patients know (not what kinds of people they are), and what things mean, is what accounts for the effectiveness of much of medical treatment. And, of course, the single most important source of knowledge and meaning for patients is their doctors. Doctors know lots of things. Many of the things that they know they are unaware of knowing (as is true for most of us in this life). But it is the depth of their convictions which conveys to patients the power of their treatments.

5   Formal factors and the meaning response

The most important aspect of any medical experience is its *content*. Whether a physician or healer prescribes aspirin or penicillin, willow bark tea or quinine, the most crucial thing is that the drug has some sort of active ingredient which interacts with the body, the immune system, a pathogen or the like, to facilitate recovery. But the content of medicines is not the only thing that counts. We have just reviewed the effect that physicians – their knowledge, their enthusiasms – can have on treatment. The *form* of medicines, their color, shape, and amount, makes a difference, too.

Meaningful pills (pink and blue ones)

In the early 1970s, several professors at the University of Cincinnati medical school devised an interesting experiment for their students (Blackwell, Bloomfield, and Buncher 1972). Fifty-seven second-year medical students agreed to participate in what they were told was a study of two new drugs. Each student would receive either a stimulant or a sedative. They were told the ordinary effects of these drugs. For example, they were told that "a sedative drug usually makes the individual feel more relaxed, calm and easy-going, but some people react by feeling drowsy, sluggish or tired. There is a tendency toward a decrease in pulse-rate, pupil size, and arterial [blood] pressure." The students were randomly divided into four groups. These groups received, respectively, one or two pink or blue tablets; the tablets were, in fact, inert. The students filled out a form describing their mood, took one another's blood pressure, took their tablets, listened to a one-hour lecture (the professors don't tell us what the lecture was about!), and then went back to the laboratory to fill out another mood rating form and to take one another's blood pressure again.

What happened? First, students who got two inert pills had more pronounced effects than those taking only one tablet. While the effects they reported ("more drowsy," "more sluggish") were generally moderate, among students who took one tablet, 6 of 119 responses were relatively severe, while among those taking two tablets, 26 of 158 responses were more severe. This is a statistically significant result (p < .005; this would occur by chance fewer than 5 times if one repeated the experiment 1,000 times).

Overall, students in the experiment felt less alert after the experiment than before. The professors attribute this to the fact that they spent an hour in class listening to that unspecified lecture. But, 66% of students who had taken blue tablets felt less alert compared to only 26% of those who had pink tablets. It is unfortunate that the professors didn't include a group of students who took no pills to see how the lecture affected *them*. But, for anyone who has ever sat through a long class, we can probably guess that the pink pills, clearly interpreted by some students as stimulants, inoculated them against some boredom!

What can we learn from this interesting experiment? First, let's consider some of the things we can eliminate. It is quite clear that the medication the students received had nothing to do with the outcome: in the first place, the tablets were designed to be inert; and, in the second place, people responded differently to the same "ingredients" depending on the color of the pills. It seems extremely unlikely that "regression to the mean" had anything to do with the results of this experiment; these students weren't sick to begin with, and although they may have been bored, since they were put into the four groups randomly, it's unlikely that the students getting blue pills were more bored to begin with than those getting pink pills. And it's unlikely that physician enthusiasm had much to do with it – presumably they were as enthusiastic about the blues as the pinks.

Clearly, the color of the pills the students took made a difference. Why? It seems pretty clear that these colors – pink and blue – have "meanings." Pinks, reds and oranges are among the colors which are called "warm" or "hot." Red is the color of stop lights, stop signs, and (traditionally, at least) fire trucks. Blue and green are "cool" colors. While one might have (or sing) the "blues," one might also listen to Jelly Roll Morton's "Red Hot Peppers" for a rather different musical experience. A study in Texas showed that red and black capsules were ranked as "strongest" while white ones were "weakest"; men had stronger preferences than did women (Sallis and Buckalew 1984). Colors are meaningful, and these meanings can affect the outcome of medical treatment.[11]

The medical students in the experiment responded exactly as this meaningful code predicts (and as the experimenters predicted). Red

---

[11] For a fascinating analysis of Western color symbolism, see Marshall Sahlins' interesting account (1976).

tablets were uppers, and blue ones were downers. Ton de Craen, a Dutch epidemiologist, has shown that this is more generally true. He and his colleagues did a study of forty-nine medicines available for sale in Holland which affect the nervous system. They found that stimulant medications tend to be marketed in red, orange or yellow tablets, while depressants or tranquilizers tend to be marketed in blue, green or purple ones (de Craen *et al.* 1996).

Soccer and the Virgin Mary

It is not always quite this simple. In a British study, people with various anxiety states responded differently to the same drug (oxazepam, or Serax, a drug similar to Valium) depending on the color of the tablet: symptoms of anxiety were more improved when the tablets were green, and symptoms of depression were more improved when the tablets were yellow (Schapira *et al.* 1970).

Two Italian studies show that there can be gender differences in these matters of color. The studies are rather complicated and a bit hard to interpret, but they seem to show that, when men and women are given blue or orange placebo sleeping pills, the women fall asleep much more quickly than the men when given blue placebos, and the duration of sleep is much longer for women given blue placebos than it is for men (Cattaneo, Lucchilli, and Filippucci 1970; Lucchelli, Cattaneo, and Zattoni 1978). In Italy, blue pills inhibit sleep in men, or promote it in women, or both, at least compared to orange pills. I am not quite sure what to make of the British study, but there may be some sense in the Italian one. In Italy, the color blue has different meanings for men and women. For women, blue is considered to be the color of the dress of the Virgin Mary. Since the Virgin is always thought of in blue, and since the Mother of God is a very reassuring and protective figure for Italian women, it seems reasonable that blue sleeping pills should be effective for them. By contrast, for Italian men, blue is the color of Azzurri, the national Italian soccer team. Blue (or azure) means success, powerful movement, strength and grace on the field, and, generally, great excitement. So it is at least plausible that blue sleeping tablets would work less well for men than for women. Orange, by contrast, is a color without strong meanings in Italian culture.[12]

---

[12] For this account of the meaning of blue in Italy, I am indebted to Lola Romanucci-Ross and her husband, John Ross, MD. Dr. Romanucci-Ross has published extensively on the anthropology of Italy. Forza Azzurri has a very cool web site at http://forzaazzurri.com/. The team slogan is "losing is not an option," not a notion conducive to a nice nap.

Another apparent exception to the notion of blue pills as being "down-ers" is the interesting case of Viagra, marketed in a pastel blue pill.[13] If anything should be displayed as an "upper," this ought to be it. The pill is prominently displayed in advertising, its lozenge shape pointing up-ward to the right. This is an interesting example of what Victor Turner has called "polysemy" – the notion that the same sign can represent dif-ferent things at different times and contexts. So, checking the Oxford English Dictionary, one finds a long list of citations following the defini-tion of the word "blue": "Affected with fear, discomfort, anxiety, etc. . . . depressed, miserable. low-spirited." But "blue" is also defined as "Inde-cent, obscene," as in the term "a blue movie," which is "libidinous." And while "blueness" may mean "indelicacy, indecency," it's also the case that "a blue-nose" is "someone who is excessively puritanical." Viagra surely partakes more of the "blue movie" than the "blue nose."

It is important to remember that, in all of these cases – the medical students from Cincinnati, and the other study subjects from Italy and Britain – the comparisons were made between people taking the same drugs, either placebo or real. The only difference was in the color. It is also important to note that these sorts of effects showed up not only when people took placebos, but also when they took real drugs. As you can see, the term "placebo effect" doesn't seem very apt here if the same thing happens whether people take placebos or active drugs. Suppose we notice that none of the sailors who eat lemons get scurvy. We call it the "lemon effect." Then we discover that no one who eats grapefruit gets scurvy. Do we still call this the "lemon effect?" We surely could, but it wouldn't be very precise.

Two is more than one

In our study with the medical students, the professors found a difference in effect not only between the colors of placebos, but also in their num-bers. Two worked better than one. Given that the pills were inert and had zero effectiveness for anything, the fact that someone took two of them shouldn't make any difference, since two times zero is still zero. But it did.

In the large series of 117 studies of treatments for ulcers, there were a number of different dosing schemes. But among all the patients in these studies, 618 patients were to take their placebos twice a day, while 1,058 were to take their placebos four times a day. After 4 weeks of taking placebos, 32.5% of the patients taking two placebos a day had no active

---

[13] Robert Hahn brought this issue to my attention, and helped solve it.

ulcers visible in the endoscope while 38.2% of the patients taking four a day had no active ulcers; that is a difference of 5.7%. This is not a big difference, but it is a statistically significant one ($\chi^2 = 5.6$, p $< .02$). There is less than one chance in 50 that this outcome is due simply to chance (Moerman 2000). In a similar study with a somewhat different set of ulcer trials, and much more sophisticated statistical techniques, Ton de Craen, a researcher in the Netherlands, has shown a larger difference than this: 36.2% of 1,504 patients taking two placebos a day were ulcer free in 4 weeks while 44.2% of 1,821 patients taking them four times a day were ulcer free; that's a difference of 8% (de Craen *et al.* 1999).

Why does this happen? Well, it seems pretty simple. What's important here is the meaning of things. When my grandson was not yet three, I asked him if he wanted one cookie or two. "Two cooks," he said, not worrying about spoiling the broth, walking away, happy as could be, with a cookie in each hand. You don't need to be a rocket scientist to know that two is more than one, or that four is more than two.

Capsules and tablets; shots and pills

These matters of color and number are matters of the *form* of medicine. There are other matters of form which make a difference as well. A Canadian study with 29 patients showed that chlordiazepoxide (Librium) was more effective against anxiety, phobias, and broken sleep when the drug was given to the patients in a capsule than when it was given as a tablet. In this study, the patients were to take pills three times per day. When they took capsules they took their pills more regularly (mean of 2.97 capsules per day) than when they took tablets (2.49 per day). Moreover, patients expressed a strong preference for the capsules: "Eleven patients requested continuation of the same treatment while receiving treatment with capsules, and on withdrawal of treatment the capsule group voiced more complaints" (Hussain and Ahad 1970). The authors conclude that both factors – patient preference and compliance – accounted for the difference in improvement.

Likewise, the route of administration of a drug (or placebo) can have a significant effect on its value. For example, it is widely recognized ("everyone knows") that shots are more powerful than pills. There is even some scientific evidence for this. In the early 1960s, a team of doctors and pharmacologists at the University of Mississippi did a very interesting experiment. They enrolled 134 patients with high blood pressure in a study of a new drug which showed promise for lowering blood pressure. They were divided into 4 groups. One group got the drug in the form of oral pills while another group got oral placebos which they took three times a day for 12 weeks. Another group received an injection of the drug, while the last group received an injection of a placebo (sterile saline solution) once every two weeks. The patients treated with pills didn't respond very well; their blood pressure dropped a small amount in both groups, but not enough to be clinically significant. The patients in groups which received injections had a much greater response. In both groups, blood pressure declined significantly for about a year (47 weeks in the group getting the drug injections, and 59 weeks in the group getting the placebo injections) whereupon it slowly went back to where it had been when the experiment began 3 years earlier. The authors conclude that the "inference to be drawn is that the parenteral [that is, injected] placebo is more effective than the oral placebo . . . [and that] more hypotensive [pressure reducing] effect is obtained from one [inert] injection every two weeks than from one [inert] tablet three times a day" (Grenfell, Briggs, and Holland 1961:129).

Taking a different approach, Ton de Craen has shown that injected placebo is more effective than oral placebo in the treatment of headache (de Craen *et al.* 2000). When the drug sumitriptan (known in the United States as Imitrex) was first introduced to treat migraine headaches, it was only available in the form of an injection; today it is still available that way, but also as tablets and nasal spray. Dr. de Craen did a meta-analysis of 35 trials, combining the data from many of them to see what the effects were. In placebo-treated patients, among those treated with a pill taken by mouth, after two hours 25.7% of patients (222 of 865) reported that their headache was better (it was gone, or mild). Of those treated with a placebo injection, 32.4% of patients (279 of 862) were better. Again, this difference is small (6.7%) but it is highly statistically significant, and could be expected to happen by chance only twice if we repeated the experiment 1000 times ($\chi^2 = 9.4$, p $= 0.002$).

What is happening here? This is one of those things which "everyone knows." The fact that we consider *all* drugs to be very powerful is probably the reason that we keep worn out medicines in the medicine cabinet in the bathroom long after their expiration dates, long after we would ever take them for anything.[14] Some of them are, however, more powerful than

---

[14] Several years ago, a student in one of my classes wanted to do a study to see just what kind of pills people thought were more powerful than others. She asked all the other students in the class to bring to her "one of each" of the pills stored in their medicine cabinets at home. Thirty students brought in so many pills that she took them home in a grocery bag. Everyone was amazed. It turned out in the study that people thought the most powerful drugs were large, multicolored capsules (especially red and white ones) and very tiny pills.

A classic (etic) account of the meaningfulness of American bathroom medicine cabinets can be found in Horace Miner's famous description of the body rituals of the

others. There are lots of things like this, things we just "know," even in the absence of evidence. We "know" that red pills are stimulants and that blue ones are depressants. We know that shots are more powerful than pills. This is the kind of thing that doctors know as well as patients (even if it isn't "true" in a particular case). We know that drugs which have to be stored in the refrigerator are more powerful than ones that can be kept in the medicine cabinet. We know that big multi-colored capsules are more powerful than white aspirin-sized tablets. We know that very tiny pills, which must be small because they have very powerful medicine in them, are stronger than aspirin-sized tablets. We know that the antiseptic medicines that we put on cuts must be red, and that wounds must be covered in order to protect them from the "air." When a sore is in a place that is hard to bandage (on a lip, for example), we cover it with grease. And we know that prescription drugs are more powerful than drugs we can buy over the counter.

There is, to my knowledge, only scientific evidence to show the first two of these are actually correct (pill color, and shots vs. pills). But the other statements are examples of the kinds of things we know which influence the way in which we interpret the meanings of our medications. And it seems that, as long as we know these things to be true, we are right.

Meaningful surgery

Another one of the things we all know is that surgery is *really* powerful. This makes excellent sense for many reasons. In a surgical procedure (what, in recent years, has come to be called "a surgery") the patient is rendered unconscious, or senseless, and a surgeon actually enters the patient's body; blood is shed (or sacrificed). The process is in its very nature dangerous. "The operation was a success, but the patient died," is a classic phrase of the surgical art, indicating the dangers surrounding even the most positive outcomes. These are powerful images. It is not surprising that they might have powerful effects on patients, and on their sickness. But, for a variety of reasons, we know very little about the meaning response in such cases.

There are very few double blind trials of surgical procedures. There are two fundamental, and closely related, reasons why this is the case. First, it is considered too dangerous. Anesthesia itself is dangerous (although much less so than as recently as the 1980s), and it is very hard to imagine that many such studies would be approved by institutional review boards,

Nacirema (Miner 1956). For a quite different (emic) take on the same situation, see J. D. Salinger's famous story "Zooey" (Salinger 1955:74–6).

or IRBs. ("IRBs" are committees of doctors, ethicists, and, often, community members who review research proposals to see that they are fair to all the patients and ethically appropriate.) But many medical procedures are dangerous; many modern drugs are very toxic and must be taken very carefully. So why is it that the dangers inherent to surgery are considered especially serious?

The reason for this, it seems to me, is rather subtle, and follows from a major difference between "medicine" and "surgery." For millennia, most drugs have been derived from some sort of natural product, usually a plant. Most of the time, there has been no obvious reason why the plant should have the effect it does on human beings. For example opium, derived from poppies, has a dramatic effect on human beings. Why would a poppy care about whether human beings get pain relief from surgery, or get high? The salicylates (precursors to aspirin, ibuprofen, and most of the other "non-steroidal anti-inflammatory drugs") are widely found in nature – in willows (the salicylates are named after the genus of willows: *Salix*), birches, and particularly in the shrubs of the genus meadowsweet (*Spiraea*), after which aspirin is named. While sometimes it is possible to speculate why plants might produce such substances (poppies are quite toxic to insects due to their opium content, and therefore are rarely eaten by them), at other times it is quite unclear. And even if it is clear what the ecological factors may be, it was still only in the 1970s that scientists discovered the *endorphins*, or "endogenous opiates" ("opiates from the inside"), which are part of the mammalian pain regulation system.[15] Generally it is the case that our experience with drugs is based on "empirical experience." Most of the time there is only very little real understanding of how drugs work. It is, for example, still not clear exactly how aspirin works, although it surely does. And so there is ample reason to devise tests which show us clearly and convincingly that some substance from whatever source *really does* stop headaches, or heal ulcers, or whatever it might be that we want to treat.

Surgery is quite different. Surgical procedures do not come from plants. They are not done for empirical reasons, but for *logical* reasons. It seems perfectly logical to put pressure on a cut or wound to stop the bleeding, to clamp down on a ruptured artery, and to forcibly remove a loose, decayed or broken tooth. Without offense, it does not require great insight or imagination to think that one might set a broken arm or remove a decayed or broken tooth. Indeed, there is evidence of chimpanzees removing the loose teeth of others using small sticks (McGrew and Tutin 1972).

---

[15] When this was discovered, many were extremely skeptical, unable to believe that the body could or would produce substances to which it might become "addicted." But it does.

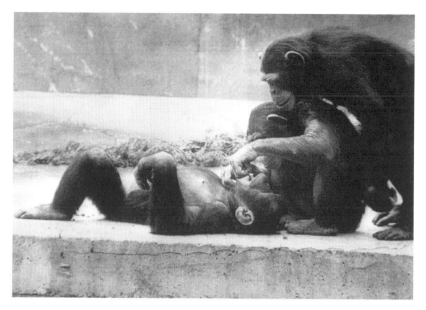

5.1   Belle removes a loose tooth from Bandit by using a small stick while Shadow looks on. Delta Primate Center, Covington, Louisiana, 1972.

While it doesn't make much sense that willow bark tea relieves headaches (since, after all, willows don't even have heads), it makes perfect sense to take out a diseased organ – an appendix, a spleen – that one might get along without; for people who are comfortable describing blood vessels as "plumbing," it makes perfect sense to put shunts around blocked arteries, as in a coronary bypass operation. As we will see, at least occasionally, it turns out that these procedures work just fine, but not necessarily because of the logic behind them. We will take a look at the logic of a very important related set of illnesses and see where it leads.

Coronary artery disease

One of the most common causes of death in the United States is myocardial infarction, or heart attack. The traditional biomedical understanding of this disease is that it is caused by *ischemia*, a lack of adequate blood flow to some region of the heart, which is in turn caused by *atherosclerosis*, which is a build-up of lipids or fatty tissues in the coronary arteries, the arteries which supply blood to the heart itself; most people have three coronary arteries, while a few have four or five. These fatty tissues, of course, are said to be due to excess cholesterol in the body, due presumably to people eating too much red meat. These lipid build-ups or atherosclerotic plaques cause lesions on the blood vessels. The heart attack is typically understood to be caused by *thrombosis*, that is, the blockage of the narrowed artery by a blood clot (a *thrombus*). The clots are said to form near sites of such fixed lesions; they are often not actually seen since, it is said, *spontaneous thrombolysis* (break down of the clots) occurs in two-thirds of cases. In any event, these clots block the artery; heart muscle, deprived of oxygenated blood, dies, creating an area in the muscle known as an *infarct* of the myocardial muscle (hence the technical name of a heart attack, a *myocardial infarction* or "MI"). The heart goes into fibrillation, and the patient dies.

In milder forms, coronary atherosclerosis is understood to lead to angina pectoris, a pressing pain beneath the sternum, which often radiates out to the left arm. The standard medical treatment for angina for the past century has been nitroglycerine tablets dissolved under the tongue. Now *there's* a powerful medicine for you! Most of us have seen the scene in the movie where someone clutches his chest, cries out "My nitro! I need my nitro!", and the bad guy tosses the pill bottle behind the couch. The poor guy dies right before our eyes, still clutching his chest. And we remember Yves Montand in the great film *Wages of Fear*, with his band of criminals, hauling truckloads of nitroglycerine over the Andes to put out an oil well fire. Our understanding of the power of medicine comes from all over. The curious thing about it is that it's not really clear why nitroglycerine stops the pain of angina attacks! It relaxes the muscles of the blood vessels, lowering blood pressure, presumably allowing more blood to get to the heart. None of this is nearly as clear as the fact that we all know how powerful nitroglycerine is!

In the past twenty years a number of important new treatments have been developed for angina. Medical treatments include beta-blockers (like propranolol, known in the US as Inderal) and calcium channel blockers (like verapamil), which seem to reduce the frequency of angina attacks. Those that still occur are treated with nitroglycerine (or a similar nitrate). But the most interesting developments in the treatment of angina have been surgical. The two most common procedures are coronary artery bypass grafting (know as CABG) and angioplasty. In CABG, arteries which are blocked by fatty deposits on the walls of the coronary arteries are, in effect, bypassed by grafting in pieces of vein or artery borrowed from other places in the body, or, sometimes, by grafting in synthetic arteries made of Dacron or similar fibers. In angioplasty, a little balloon is threaded up to the coronary arteries and inflated. This expands the artery, allowing more blood flow to the heart. Given these theories of blocked "pipes" (that's what heart surgeons call arteries), these procedures, easily visualized when you look at a bit of rusted plumbing from the laundry tub, make very good sense.

But there's more to it than that. These "pipes" are part of thinking, knowing people. Angina pectoris, a grave and dangerous symptom of serious underlying pathology, is, it turns out, highly responsive not only to nitrates and beta blockers but also to inert treatment as well.[16] This seems quite surprising as the theory of sclerotic arteries and blood clots – rusty plumbing – would seem to leave little place for such unlikely findings.

Here is one example of an unlikely finding. In a European double blind, randomized trial of two different drugs for treating angina lasting six months, 35 patients were treated only with placebos and nitroglycerine for the six-month period. At the beginning of the study, these patients had an average of 10.3 angina attacks per week, and, on average, they took 10.6 nitroglycerine tablets. After admission to the study, the patients' dose of placebo was adjusted for a period of eight weeks until it was satisfactory (as was done for all the patients in the trial). Then, this dosage was continued for another four months. Twenty-seven of the 35 placebo-treated patients (77% of them) showed substantial improvements over the period. Overall, the average number of angina attacks dropped from 10.3 to 2.4 per week; the number of nitroglycerine tablets used dropped from 10.6 to 2.1. Exercise time until an angina attack increased from 9.3 to 10.2 minutes (Boissel *et al.* 1986). Given the theory of rusty pipes, this is a very surprising result. It seems unlikely that these people would simply have gotten better had they stayed at home and had no treatment at all; "most of the patients had severely limited functional status . . . [and] most had been previously treated: 21 with long acting nitrates, 18 with beta-blocking agents, 9 with calcium-channel blockers. Only 1 received no treatment prior to entry into the study." These were people who were quite sick, and there was little reason to expect that they would get better without treatment. But, with inert treatment in a clinical trial, they did get better.

The logic of this theory of rusty pipes has had a long history. Several indirect revascularization techniques which involved rerouting various arteries were developed in the 1930s by Beck and in the 1940s by Vineburg (Meade 1961:480–515). Although Beck's procedure attained modest popularity, the first widely used surgical approach to angina was the bilateral internal mammary artery ligation (BIMAL). The internal mammary (or thoracic) arteries arise from the subclavian artery high in the chest

---

[16] Bienenfeld's review of the placebo effect in cardiovascular disease in the *American Heart Journal* is particularly thorough and interesting (Bienenfeld, Frishman, and Glasser 1996).

and descend just inside the front wall of the chest, ultimately supplying blood throughout the chest and viscera. Following anatomical research by Fieschi, an Italian surgeon, which indicated connections between various ramifications of these arteries and the coronary circulation, several other Italian surgeons developed a procedure in which the arteries were ligated (tied off) below the point where these branches presumably diverged to the heart in order to enhance this flow and supplement the blood supply. The operation was first performed in the United States by Robert Glover and J. Roderick Kitchell in the late 1950s (Glover 1957; Kitchell, Glover and Kyle 1958). It was quite simple, and since the arteries were not deep in the body, could be performed under local anesthesia. The physicians reported symptomatic improvement (ranging from slight to total) in 68% of their first sample of fifty patients, in a two- to six-month follow-up. The operation quickly gained some popularity.

The problem is that no one else believed that there *was* any real connection between these arteries and the heart! So, shortly after these reports appeared, two different surgical teams at two American medical centers – one from Kansas City under the direction of E. Grey Dimond (Dimond, Kittle, and Crockett 1960) and the other in Seattle under Leonard Cobb (Cobb *et al.* 1959) – did double blind trials of the procedure. In each case, the surgeon learned only while in the operating room which patients were to have the complete operation and which were to receive "sham surgery." Those patients received the complete operation, but the arteries were not ligated. In both studies, the patients were followed for at least six months after the surgery by cardiologists who were unaware of which patients had received the ligations and which had not. In one of the studies (Seattle) the patients were told that the operation was experimental, but they were not informed that some of them would get the sham surgery. In the Kansas City study, it is not clear from the publication just what the patients were told; it does say that the patients did not know which procedure they had received (suggesting that they knew there were two possibilities). This seems not to have made any difference anyway. In both studies, most of the patients were much better after surgery regardless of whether they had the full operation or the sham surgery. Table 5.1 indicates the outcomes of the two studies and shows the combined outcome.

In both cases, patients experienced significant subjective improvement; that is, they reported that they had substantially less pain than before the surgery. This was true regardless of whether or not they had the full procedure (67% substantial improvement) or the sham procedure (82% substantial improvement). In the Seattle study, "need for nitroglycerine was uniformly decreased." In the Kansas city study, the average

Table 5.1. *Outcome of actual and sham surgery for angina pectoris; amount of subjective improvement*

	Actual surgery				Sham surgery			
Improvement	Seattle	K. C.	Total	Percent	Seattle	K. C.	Total	Percent
Substantial	5	9	14	67%	5	5	10	83%
Slight	3	4	7	33%	2	0	2	17%
Total	8	13	21		7	5	12	

number of nitroglycerine tablets taken per week dropped 34% in patients with the full operation and 42% in patients with the sham operation. In both studies, patients were, on average, able to exercise longer before an angina attack. In neither study were there substantial changes in electrocardiogram readings, although one Seattle patient with striking abnormalities before surgery had none afterwards. He received the sham surgery.

It is hard to know how to account for the substantial improvement in these patients. Whatever the truth may be about the alleged connection between the internal mammary arteries and the coronary arteries (it doesn't show up anywhere in my *Gray's Anatomy!*), it doesn't really matter; in these two studies, the patients with the sham procedure did as well (maybe even a bit better) than those with the complete procedure. But for people willing to trust their surgeons and doctors, this is a pretty compelling operation. The notion that your heart is starved for blood makes pretty good sense. And the notion that we can, by shutting off the flow of blood down one pipe, enhance the flow into another pipe – sort of like what happens in the bathroom sink when you turn off the shower – makes very good sense. One patient in the Kansas City study, when asked if he felt better, said, "Yes. Practically immediately I felt better. I felt I could take a deep breath... I figure I'm about 95 percent better. I was taking five nitros a day before surgery. In the first five weeks following, I have taken a total of twelve." This patient's arteries were not ligated (Dimond, Kittle, and Crockett 1960:484). But he did have two scars on his chest, and he had an explanation that made sense (unless he was an aficionado of *Gray's Anatomy*). He had all the elements of meaning which he needed.

It is also interesting to notice that the improvements here – 67% and 82% – are much the same as the improvements reported by Boissel – 77% – in the six-month placebo treatment of angina mentioned earlier, a good deal higher than that usually attributed to inert treatment.

There are other, similar, cases where one can make similar arguments, although not from double blind trials. As I have already noted, the surgical procedure known as coronary artery bypass grafting (CABG) is one of the most common surgical approaches to angina pectoris today. It is not clear how many such procedures may be done in a year, but various estimates suggest that it is about 600,000 per year in the United States. At roughly $50,000 each, this is a $30 billion dollar-a-year industry. The approach with CABG is different from the BIMAL. Here, the idea is to take another piece of blood vessel (sometimes the saphenous vein from the leg, and sometimes a piece of the same internal mammary artery which was ligated in the BIMAL) and to place shunts around the regions in the coronary arteries which seem to be blocked by the fatty atherosclerotic deposits. This should allow more blood to get to the heart and should stop the anginal pain caused by this ischemia. This procedure is far more invasive than the BIMAL. The patient is anaesthetized, and the surgeon performs a median sternotomy (that's formal surgery language; informally, surgeons say they "crack the chest"). The heart is stopped and the patient is attached to a heart-lung machine.[17] An artery or vein is "harvested" and then used to make the shunts across the blocked portions of the coronary arteries; the occluded areas are "bypassed."

This is one of the most successful forms of surgery ever developed. The logic is perfectly clear, and 90 percent of patients find themselves pain free after it is over. But that was the case with the BIMAL patients, too, and with the patients taking the drugs subsequently shown not to be more effective than placebo. And, unsurprisingly, CABG has never been subjected to a double blind trial comparing it to sham surgery.[18]

There is every reason to believe that, today, CABG works more or less the way its defenders propose. Without doubt, the operation relieves pain in 80% or 90% of patients who have it. Moreover, their electrocardiogram readings become more normal and their exercise tolerance increases. This, however, was not always so. In the early days of the operation, during the 1970s, while many patients experienced the same pain relief of more recent times, many did not show the increase in exercise tolerance, and they didn't show the improvement in electrocardiogram readings. Analyzing the situation in the late 1970s, one group of researchers suggested that, after the operation, the ischemia (restricted blood flow) persisted, even though the pain was not present (Bulkley and

---

[17] In recent years, some surgeons have developed techniques for applying the shunts on the beating heart, not stopping it, and not using the heart-lung machine (Murkin *et al.* 1999). This is, as yet, still relatively rare, but it is becoming more common.

[18] Although a highly regarded thoracic surgeon once argued *vigorously* with me saying that there had been such a study. An exhaustive search of the medical literature reveals that there hasn't.

Ross 1978). These doctors suggested that this could have been due to several things: the heart could have been "denervated" – that is, the operation could have inadvertently destroyed nerve fibers to the heart, so that pain couldn't be felt any more; or the operation could have killed some previously living heart tissue which would, thereafter, be insensitive to pain. They also suggest that the pain reduction could have been due to the placebo effect.

Another team of investigators soon after reported something similar. It is often the case (probably more in the early days of the operation than now) that grafts around occluded regions of the heart muscle simply don't "take," or become "patent." Yet these patients with unsuccessful bypasses, in whom it is hard to imagine how the blood flow to the heart could be much improved, showed the same high levels of pain relief as did those with patent graphs (see, for example, Valdes *et al.* 1979).

These problems have largely been solved by now with significant improvements in surgical technique: grafts last for many years, and blood flow to the heart after CABG is clearly increased. But this doesn't change the fact that the pain relief occurred in those early patients with significantly less effective surgery.

Placebo pacemakers

There is additional evidence of meaningful responses to surgery. In a study in Sweden done in the late 1990s, 81 people with "hypertrophic cardiomyopathy" were operated on and given pacemakers. Hypertrophic cardiomyopathy is a condition in which the heart muscle thickens abnormally; it can be a fairly benign condition, but it can also be very serious, causing sudden death. It is treated with a range of options including beta-blockers or other medications, heart valve surgery, or by installing pacemaker. In the Swedish study, half the pacemakers which were installed were, in effect, not turned on. While the patients with working pacemakers did better overall than those whose implants had not been turned on, the latter were doing much better after three months than they were when the study began. Unfortunately, this study did not have an untreated control group; but unfortunately, too, it is not a condition which simply goes away of its own accord very often. Patients with turned-off pacemakers experienced significantly less chest pain, shortness of breath, dizziness, and heart palpitations, and they experienced an improvement in cognitive functioning (thinking) after three months. The authors of the study concluded: "The placebo effect of pacemaker implantation appears to be substantial. Although it is hard to evaluate, it must be taken into account . . . " (Linde *et al.* 1999). (As per my standard commentary:

there are no placebos here; this is not a placebo effect, but a meaning response.)

"Bloodlines" and lasers

"Bloodlines are paths that allow oxygen-rich blood to saturate oxygen-starved heart tissue. One laser can create bloodlines: the CO_2 Heart Laser™." Well, that's what it says on the website of the company that makes the laser, PLC Medical Systems, Inc.[19]

"Transmyocardial laser revascularization" (TMR) is the latest whistle in the surgical approach to angina. A company spokesperson told me that they estimated they were approaching a total of 6,000 procedures worldwide (in spring 2000), explaining that, after the procedure was covered by Medicare, it quickly gained widespread acceptance as a treatment for angina by the medical world (Floody 2000).

What kind of operation is this? In TMR, an incision is made in the side of the chest between two ribs. The outer layer of the heart (the pericardium) is removed, and the heart muscle (the myocardium) is exposed. A laser (several different types are used) is touched to the surface of the heart, and a laser beam is fired into the heart, presumably to make a channel through the heart. Usually thirty to fifty such channels are made. The idea is that this will make a sort of substitute artery, a "bloodline" in the terms of one company, through which blood will flow providing oxygen-rich blood directly to the heart muscle. The pericardium is replaced, and the incision in the chest is closed.

Interestingly enough, the origins of this operation lie in some experiments done in the 1960s where a doctor, making an analogy with the way reptile hearts work (reptile hearts don't get blood delivered via arteries, but the blood simply suffuses from the ventricles into the heart muscle itself through cavities called "sinusoids"), decided simply to make such channels using acupuncture needles! Subsequently some other researchers decided to try using lasers to do the same thing (for a clear history of the procedure, see Kantor *et al.* 1999). By the mid-1990s, a number of fairly large trials had been carried out. The procedure was reserved for people who were not healthy enough to be treated by the standard techniques (CABG, angiography), and who had very serious, unstable end-stage angina – that is, for very sick people. The results were quite remarkable: success rates were in the range of 75% to 90%.

---

[19] Fall, 2001: http://www.plcmed.com/intro.htm; remember that websites change frequently. This is a very snazzy site with dramatic graphics, worth looking at as an example of how private companies can create medical meaning. The website also refers to bloodlines with the less dramatic term "channels."

"Success" was defined as very significant improvement in pain and functioning. Angina is characterized in several ways; one uses the Canadian Cardiovascular Society system which sorts angina into four classes.[20] Successful improvement in these studies required a two-stage improvement; that's a lot for such very sick people.

The problem is that no one really knows how or why this operation "works." The "bloodlines" close up in a matter of hours, and there is no evidence that the myocardial blood flow actually increases by the best type of evidence, perfusion imaging (Landolfo *et al.* 1999). The analogy with the reptile heart simply doesn't work; mammalian hearts just don't have the reptilian sinusoids. So what *does* happen? Some say that the laser beams disrupt the nerves of the heart and denervate the affected areas (Al-Sheikh *et al.* 1999), but others seem to show pretty conclusively that this is not the case (Hirsch *et al.* 1999). There is some reason to believe that the scarring process may lead to the creation of some new blood vessels ("angiogenesis"), but there is no clear evidence that this has any effect on angina.

So, what's left? A number of people who have looked at the situation suggest that, by analogy with the bilateral internal mammary artery ligation, this may be due to the placebo effect (for example, Kantor *et al.* 1999; Lange and Hillis 1999). There are minimal improvements in the objective measures of heart disease; but for patients, the most important thing is not objective measures of anything, but whether or not they can climb stairs, lift their grandchildren, or mow the lawn.

More recently, Dr. Martin Leon and a group of colleagues from across the US enrolled 300 patients in a placebo-controlled trial of a related procedure similar in form to angioplasty. A laser catheter was inserted in the femoral artery and threaded up into the left ventricle; the laser pulses were administered from inside out; this requires much less invasive surgery. These patients were very sick:

- all were rated as Class III or IV on the four-stage Canadian scale;
- 90% had previously had bypass surgery;
- 65% had previously had heart attacks;
- all had had angioplasty within the previous four months;
- yet they were relatively young people, averaging about 62 years in age.

Patients were randomly assigned to one of three groups: a high-dose group (twenty to twenty-five laser punctures); a low-dose group (ten to fifteen laser punctures); or a mock procedure with only simulated laser treatment. All three groups displayed similar impressive improvement six

[20] In Class I, ordinary activity (walking, climbing stairs) does not cause angina, but rapid, strenuous and prolonged exertion may. In Class IV, people are unable to carry out any activity without discomfort; anginal pain can occur at rest, while sitting in a chair.

months after surgery on all objective and subjective measures which were observed. Exercise tolerance was increased in all three groups. The percentage of patients who improved two or more classes on the Canadian scale ranged from 25% (high dose) to 33% (placebo) to 39% (low dose). Frequency of angina declined, and physical functioning and disease perception scores increased, in all three groups. None of the modest differences between the three groups were statistically significant (Leon et al. 2000).

Recall that these were very sick people, many of them in their fifties or younger. They all showed remarkable improvement regardless of whether there were any channels placed in the heart muscles.

In the early 1990s, before the FDA had approved this laser treatment, Dr. Alan G. Johnson wrote an article titled "Surgery as a placebo" in *The Lancet* (a leading British medical journal), and he noted that "electrical machines have great appeal to patients, and recently anything with the word 'laser' attached to it has caught the imagination" (Johnson 1994). It may be worth suggesting that doctors, as well as patients, find their imaginations fired by lasers (surely more than by acupuncture needles)!

Lumbar disk herniation

These kinds of effects can be seen in areas other than cardiology and thoracic surgery. As I noted at the beginning, there aren't many cases where we can actually demonstrate the effects of placebo surgery since randomized controlled trials of such procedures are quite rare. But there are some similar situations which, carefully interpreted, can yield similar conclusions. In 1972, researcher Erik Spangfort did a very comprehensive analysis of all the surgical operations carried out for suspected lumbar disc herniation between 1959 and 1965 in Sweden, a total of 2,503 operations. The main symptoms of "slipped disc" was some form of sciatica (pain running down the leg along the sciatic nerve) often accompanied by persistent back pain. The diagnosis is based largely on analysis of x-rays of the back, plus a series of additional neurological tests. The surgery involves exposing the disc and "removing all loose fragments of disc tissue, . . . and to excise degenerated tissue from the interior of the intervertebral space without attempting to remove the total disc" (Spangfort 1972:7). In the course of his review, Spangfort noted that 346 patients with all the appropriate symptoms and signs turned out not to have degenerated discs after all. He called these, variously, "negative explorations" or "negative operations." In these cases of what turned out to be "exploratory surgery," nothing was done to the discs, and the patients' wounds were simply closed. With these patients one would imagine that, since the healthy disc was not, apparently, the cause of their pain, and since nothing was done to them except sufficient surgery to observe the disc, there would be no particular outcome to the procedure. But Spangfort reports that, six months after surgery, 37% of these patients had complete relief of their sciatic pain; another 133 (38.4%) had partial relief of their sciatica. Three quarters of these "sham surgery" patients were improved. Only 85 patients (25%) were the same or worse as they were before surgery. He also looked at the effect on "persistent low back pain," but this time one year after surgery; 43% of patients with "negative operations" had no back pain a year later.

One researcher has commented on Spangfort's findings by saying "There is no known therapeutic effect of surgical exploration of the lumbar spine" (Turner *et al.* 1994:610). Unfortunately, we have no way of knowing what the surgeons told their patients after this "unsuccessful" surgery. We might guess that they were told that their discs were (now?) in fine shape and they would just have to wait and see. And up to three quarters of them were substantially better.

Ménière's disease

Ménière's disease is a very unpleasant and potentially debilitating condition affecting the inner ear. On unpredictable occasions, someone with this condition can experience severe dizziness, tinnitus or loud roaring in the ears, hearing loss, and pain or pressure in the ear. The part of the ear known as the "labyrinth" is filled with liquid; as you move your head, the liquid stimulates nerve endings which send signals to the brain to indicate the nature of your movements, so you can maintain your balance. Should this fluid ("endolymph") increase in quantity, causing pressure on the labyrinth, it stops working properly, causing the dizziness and other symptoms. The cause of the increase in the fluid is unknown. There are many treatments for the condition, none of them foolproof. In the 1970s several surgical approaches were developed for Ménière's disease (which is named after a French doctor who first described it in the mid-nineteenth century; it is now also called "endolymphatic hydrops"). A common procedure was to insert a small tube into the affected region so the excessive fluid could be drained away. In 1981, several Danish physicians published the results of a controlled clinical trial of this surgical procedure. They treated thirty people with Ménière's disease; in fifteen, they installed the drainage tubes while in the remaining fifteen they did a mastoidectomy, a fairly common procedure for ear diseases, but not in any way considered to be a treatment for Ménière's disease (Thomsen *et al.* 1981). They reported that, a year later, there were no differences between the two groups, and 70% of the patients in both groups were much improved. This improvement in both groups, which they attributed to the placebo effect, was still evident nine years later (Bretlau *et al.* 1989).[21] People can respond to inert treatment, including surgical treatments, for a long time.

Conclusions

What can we conclude from this review of formal factors in the meaning response? Large pills work better than middle-sized pills. Blue pills make better sleeping pills than pills of other colors (except for Italian soccer fans). Four inert pills work better than two. Pills work fine, but shots work better. Surgery works better yet, even if it sometimes doesn't actually do anything to the person being operated on. High-powered machines with snappy names, especially ones that remind us of video games, may be at the top of the heap. The *form* of medical treatment, not just its *content*, can have a dramatic effect on human wellbeing.

And notice something else. In the previous chapter, I presented a range of evidence to show that doctors were more important than patients in generating meaning responses. This view is generally quite the reverse of the standard view which most people have, where people (or at least medical professionals) still believe – against all the evidence – that patients are the source of these responses. In that case, the general wisdom, the common sense, is opposite to what the evidence shows. In this chapter, I have looked at the form of medicine, its shapes and colors: I have shown that pink pills work differently than blue ones, that two inert pills work better than one, that capsules work better than tablets, and that shots work better than pills (even if both are inert); and I have shown that inert surgery works nearly as well as real surgery. This is not in any obvious way the "opposite" of common sense; it simply defies common sense. In either case, we learn to be wary of our common sense when we think about medicine.

---

[21] More recently, other researchers have re-evaluated the data reported by the original authors at the one-year follow-up using newer statistical techniques, finding the drainage tube operation to be more effective than the mastoidectomy (Welling and Nagaraja 2000); regardless, over 70% of the patients with the sham treatment still felt the operation had produced good results nine years later.

6 Knowledge and culture; illness and healing

> The biomedical model of disease is so pervasive that we often fail to see it as such but view it as reality. Questioning this model is like asking whether a goldfish knows it is in water.
>
> O'Boyle, 1993

These sorts of things – from blue pills to lasers – are all things which we "know," even though, like the goldfish, we may not realize that we know them. Much of our knowledge of the world is not an elicitation of what "is," but rather it is a construction laid atop the world of experience. This is a very difficult concept for many people to grasp. The world that we see and experience seems so palpable and true, and our conceptualizations are so deeply entwined among themselves, that it just seems fantasy to say that the reality I perceive is largely metaphor and construction and is largely projected onto (rather than observed in) the world.[22] These things are generally true, and they are true for many matters of health and medicine. This chapter may not convince a skeptic. But it may encourage the enquiring, and its goal is to make the strangeness of the placebo effect and the meaning response somewhat less strange. The price to be paid is that everything else gets rather more strange. *C'est la vie.*

Proper meals, clothing, pills

In the United States, we "know" that one eats (or, ought to eat) three meals a day[23]; if you don't, your mother gets mad at you. Those meals come in an ordered set which can be characterized as "breakfast, lunch, and DINNER" – two subordinate elements and a dominant one which

---

[22] Two sources which can help you understand this perspective better are *The Social Construction of Reality* (Berger and Luckmann 1967) and *Metaphors We Live By* (Lakoff and Johnson 1980).

[23] My discussion of food habits is inspired by Mary Douglas' and Marshall Sahlins' various writings about the subject (Douglas 1966; Sahlins 1978). The size and complexity of the problem is hinted at by the scope of Claude Levi-Strauss' four-volume *Mythologiques* which deals essentially with the origins of cooking, table-manners, and so on (*The Raw and the Cooked*, *The Origin of Table Manners*, and *From Honey to Ashes*, for example).

I might represent by a little formula, "A + 2b." In addition, many of the meals we eat can be characterized by the same formula, so a classic dinner might include "ENTREE, salad, and dessert." And the main part of the meal might include "mashed potatoes, peas, and MEAT LOAF." A salad might contain "LETTUCE, tomato, and dressing," while the dressing might be made of "vinegar, mustard, and OIL." Our utensils might be "a FORK, a knife, and a spoon." A simpler lunch might consist of a peanut butter and jelly sandwich, while breakfast might consist of bacon, eggs and toast (applying the formula in these cases is an exercise left to the reader). To see the "A + 2b" formula in all its richness, look at the pictures on the tv-dinners at a supermarket some time.

Now the interesting thing about this is that while we all "know" this formula, and we all know how to apply it, most of us don't really know that we know it. And no one "discovered" that he or she should eat this way; rather it's the other way around: we eat this way because it's what we know, because it's the "right" way to do things. Such knowledge is the basis of the moral structure of human relationships in a society (we know we are dealing with morality when we are talking about things being "right"). One doesn't discover something like a food formula by studying nutrition (such study might lead to the "four food groups" or the "food triangle"), but by studying culture and human behavior. You can learn a good deal about nutrition and "food triangles" by studying rats. However, you can learn nothing about the "right" kind of food from such research.

This is similarly the case with the things which we allow on our table, which we define as edible. In ordinary American life, it's cows and pigs, but not dogs or horses. This seems like the natural order of things – some things are edible, and some are not. But cows are forbidden for Hindus, as are pigs for Jews, while dogs are a favorite item on the menu for many Native American and Asian peoples, and horse is a special delicacy in France, the basis for "steak tartare" among other dishes. Many have tried to make functional arguments about these choices, to say that some things literally are edible and others are not (Harris 1985), but such attempts always founder on the data – one imagines that it could be proven that every culture has some item of food which it most esteems, and that if we look closely enough, we will find another group which considers it an abomination. Some years ago, the Food and Drug Administration, in an effort to improve the "cleanliness" of the nation's food supply, applied more stringent standards to the amount of insect debris which could be legally contained in flour (insects are, in the United States, an abomination, the essence of the "unclean", although they are eaten in many other parts of the world). This action reduced the protein value of the flour; but it was "clean"! One entomologist has argued that, in many tropical and subtropical countries where insects have long been a traditional food, the Western bias against eating insects "has had an adverse impact, resulting in a gradual reduction in the use of insects without replacement of lost nutrition and other benefits" (DeFoliart 1999).

Note that such a cultural element can have a perceptible biological consequence. For example, one might easily make a dinner of "rice, pea pods, and a PORK CHOP." But one might also order shredded pork and pea pods served over rice in a Chinese restaurant. The ingredients could be exactly the same in both dinners. But how often do Americans say, two hours later, that they are really hungry after "eating Chinese?" Why? It's not because they didn't get enough food; what was missing was the formula. Such a structure transforms the simple act of eating into the meaningful human act of dining. German has two words for the verb "to eat": *fressen* is eating by animals, while *essen* is eating by people. Thus, human eating has two dimensions – the nutritional and the meaningful.

One might well argue that just about everything people do has such a dual nature. If I speak to you, saying "I love you," regardless of what else we might think about it, I am exhaling in the process. Talking is a way we make breathing meaningful (so is singing, whistling a happy tune, humming to myself, or playing jazz on a saxophone). In most languages, talking occurs on the exhale; but in some African languages people modulate their inhaling with clicks and slides that are particularly melodious. Most people in the world wear clothes which might protect them from the elements, from cold and rain. But clothing is also always meaningful: it is very commonly the case that children dress differently than adults, and that men dress differently than women; the notion that clothing is *only* functional is easily belied by, say, a tuxedo or a bikini.

Such meaning changes things and makes things happen. As I say "I love you," I eliminate carbon dioxide from my chest; but I also shape and form our relationship. When I put on my most powerful suit before going to an interview, I am protected from the wind and I feel empowered. I put on a white lab coat with a stethoscope hanging out of my pocket before going out onto the hospital ward even though there is no chance I will be in a laboratory, and even though I may be working on the orthopedic ward where there is little need to listen to lungs. My lab coat is a uniform, an indicator of my status in the hospital, not anything practical (Blumhagen 1979). I once observed a senior professor in a medical school come breezing in eight or ten minutes late for a lecture after lunch. He made a hundred students wait another three minutes while he changed from his tweed jacket to his lab coat before beginning his lecture. First things first.

The situation is, obviously, very much like taking an aspirin tablet where the effect is a combination of the actions of the acetylsalicylic acid, and of the meaning of the pill and, perhaps, its brand name. Medicine is not the only meaningful kind of human behavior – far from it. It is only one aspect of a broadly human reality where everything that we do, like it or not, intended or otherwise, is impregnated with meaning which constructs our very lives.

Much of the meaning of medicine, of the meaning response (and in the narrowest sense, the placebo effect), is a cultural phenomenon engaged in a complex interplay on the meanings of disease and illness. The modern triumph of a universalist biology tends to blind us to the dramatic variation in the ways that people experience their own physiology based on who they are and what they know.

Knowing acupuncture and analgesia

While meaning is always important in medicine, it is interesting that, sometimes, doctor and patient may not share the same system of meaning. Traditional Chinese Medicine is based in large part on the manipulation of *chi* (usually translated as "energy") using a combination of herbal treatments, acupuncture and so on (Beinfield and Korngold 1991). Acupuncture, in particular, has become quite popular in the West (Eisenberg *et al.* 1998). Yet few Western patients know much about *chi* or its manipulation, and most would have difficulty fitting such knowledge into their school-based understanding of physiology – nerves, blood vessels, and so on. Their knowledge of Oriental medicine in general and acupuncture in particular is probably based on their watching Bill Moyers on television, where they may have learned that "acupuncture works," although for no evident reasons. Claire Cassidy has found that, even after six months of acupuncture care, American patients still have a very sketchy understanding of the system, at least in terms authentic to Oriental medicine, yet they are very enthusiastic about their care which they deem extremely effective (Cassidy 1998). What westerners know about acupuncture is, generally, that they think it works. But more than that is required for effectiveness.

One of the most effective single uses for acupuncture is in preventing nausea and vomiting after surgery. This is a common and, potentially, very serious problem, as people who are still very groggy after anesthesia can choke on their own vomit. A large body of work, most of it following pioneering studies by J. W. Dundee in Ireland, has shown that acupuncture of one point on the forearm known as "P-6" or "Neiguan," can dramatically reduce this nausea and vomiting (Dundee *et al.* 1989). The P-6 or Neiguan acupuncture point can be found this way: take three fingers on one hand, and place the third (ring) finger across the inside of the wrist; the P-6 point is about where the index finger crosses the space between two tendons on the lower arm which you can feel with that finger.

Many studies have shown that such acupuncture is more effective than no treatment, or sham acupuncture treatment of some sort, for nausea and vomiting.

Perhaps the most interesting aspect of this issue is that there is evidence to indicate that, regardless of *what* it is that they know about acupuncture, people apparently have to *be aware* of having it in order for it to be effective. Andrew Vickers did a meta-analysis of thirty-three controlled trials of this procedure. While P-6 acupuncture was only equal to, or less effective than, the control condition (sham or misplaced acupuncture) in four studies where the treatment was administered to the patients after they had been anaesthetized, in twenty-seven of the remaining twenty-nine studies – when patients were awake and aware when the acupuncture was given – the treatment was better than controls (Vickers 1996). In order for this treatment to work (or at least for it to work well enough to be better than the control), you have to know that you have had it, and to experience the having of it! If you get the acupuncture, but don't know it, or, if you experience acupuncture, but it is a fake product (misplaced, or with a sham needle), it won't work. Knowledge makes a difference and somehow activates (real, but not fake) acupuncture.

In another study, this one done in France, a group of forty-nine cancer patients with moderate pain were admitted to a study of the effects of naproxen, a non-steroidal anti-inflammatory drug similar to (but somewhat stronger than) aspirin and ibuprofen. Twenty of these patients were given a pill on their first morning in the hospital without being told anything about it. Among these patients, half were given naproxen, while half were given a matching placebo. The next day, the treatments were switched, and the patients who had previously had naproxen now got a placebo, and vice-versa. The remaining twenty-four patients were treated differently. Before they received any drugs, they were given detailed information about the experiment, and were told about the placebos and the naproxen. Six of them declined to participate in the study because they didn't want to get a placebo treatment; eighteen participated.

The results of the study are very interesting. In both study groups, naproxen worked better than placebo in treating cancer pain. But both naproxen and placebo worked substantially better for the patients who had been told about the experiment than they did for the patients in the dark about the procedure. Indeed, in the informed patients, the placebos worked much better than did the naproxen in the uninformed patients. The experimenters put it this way: "Information . . . induces changes in therapeutic efficacy" (Bergmann *et al.* 1994).

In the previous case, people who were unconscious couldn't get the benefits of the acupuncture treatment. In this case, a discussion about the fact of getting drugs, and even of the possibility of getting an inert drug, increased the effectiveness of both the drug and the placebo. Knowing what's going on, experiencing treatment both physically and verbally, makes a difference.

Knowing things is not simply a matter of being awake, of talking with your doctor about an experiment, or experiencing acupuncture. Knowing things is also a complex human and cultural phenomenon. In different places in the world, people know different things; experiencing the world with a different language, different history and social institutions, and different customs means that, comparing one place to another we find significantly different fabrics of meaning woven from these different strands. It does not mean that all Chinese think alike, or that all Navajos on the one hand or Americans on the other see the world in identical ways. But there are dramatic differences in the patterns of thought on which individuality, difference and agency are formed. This is often complicated for people to deal with. How can people "know" one thing in one place, and a different thing in another place? One "knows" the "truth." Can there be two truths? Well, yes. (Indeed, there can be many more than two.)

We have seen in several contexts how the things that people know and understand shape the way that medicine has its effects. People "know," for example that a particular kind of aspirin is really good because they have seen it advertised on television. But much of the knowledge that people have of the world does not have such an explicit source or origin. Much of what we know we simply grow up with, as matters of culture; there are ways of knowing the world which are simply different for French or German or Italian or Inuit or Maori or American people. Different foods seem edible and, are prepared in different ways and eaten at different times of day; different languages shape experience differently; different political histories shape different views of the appropriate relationships between friends, family, employees, and so on. This is the ordinary substance of anthropology. Culture is a hard word to define, but it's not uncommon for definitions to include something about "ways of knowing the world." It seems as if these different ways of knowing the world can show up in the different effectiveness of medication and of meaning in matters of health.

There is an important qualification on this argument: It is important to note that "country" is not a very close indicator of culture. In France, for example, Normandy in the north is very different from Provence in the south, and Paris is very different from Strasbourg or Marseilles. And the variation in style of life, diet, and language in Brazil will dwarf the differences in France. So to say that France, or Brazil, represent "cultures" is clearly a significant oversimplification. On the other hand, at least in this context, these sorts of medical studies are almost always done in national laboratories or university hospitals. Patients will be relatively cosmopolitan, and relatively urban; it is extremely unlikely that any indigenous people of the Brazilian rainforests will be in these patient groups. Such studies are also often multi-center trials; a French study of ulcer treatment that I will describe later in this chapter included patients from ten hospitals in major cities across France including Paris, Lyon, Tour, Rennes, Toulouse, and Marseilles. Such trials might yield something more generically "French" than would a similar trial carried out only in Paris or Toulouse.[24] Regardless, it is clear that using countries as proxies for culture is risky at best. However, until more finely grained research can be carried out, it is the best we can do.

Menopause, estrogen and culture

So, in the cases just described, people who knew things that others didn't (because the latter had been under anesthesia) responded differently; and people who knew they were getting anesthesia needed less than those who didn't know in order to get the same relief. In the next few cases I will describe, there are differences in what appear to be matters of biology and medicine which can be attributed to cultural patterns (recognizing the caveat of "nation" and "culture") where the different ways different people know the world influence biology.

The seventeenth edition of *The Merck Manual* (a widely utilized medical textbook) defines menopause as "Physiologic cessation of menses due to decreasing ovarian function" (Beers and Berkow 1999). This purely biological definition is followed by a description of symptoms:

Symptoms of the climacteric range from nonexistent to severe. Hot flushes (flashes) and sweating secondary to vasomotor instability affect 75% of women. Most have hot flushes for >1 yr, and 25 to 50% for >5 yr. The woman feels warm or hot and may perspire, sometimes profusely. The skin, especially of the head and neck, becomes red and warm. The flush, which may last from 30 sec to 5 min, may be followed by chills.

The explanation for these phenomena is, again, purely biological, and is phrased in terms of an inevitable change in hormonal activity:

Menopause occurs naturally at an average age of 50 to 51 yr in the USA.[25] As ovaries age, response to pituitary gonadotropins (follicle-stimulating hormone

[24] It may be worth noting that published reports of clinical studies often simply do not mention where the work was done. This makes sense if the researchers see location as irrelevant, if human biology is universal.

[25] The fifteenth edition of the *Manual*, published in 1987, says that "natural menopause occurs at an average of 49 to 50 yr" and omits the phrase "in the USA." It is possible that even the authors of the *Merck Manual* are beginning to realize that biology is cultural!

[FSH] and luteinizing hormone [LH]) decreases, initially resulting in shorter follicular phases (thus, shorter menstrual cycles), fewer ovulations, decreased progesterone production, and more irregularity in cycles. Eventually, the follicle fails to respond and does not produce estrogen. Without estrogen feedback, circulating levels of LH and FSH rise substantially. Circulating levels of estrogens and progesterone are markedly reduced. The androgen androstenedione is reduced by half, but testosterone decreases only slightly because the stroma of the postmenopausal ovary continues to secrete substantial amounts (as does the adrenal gland). Androgens are converted to estrogens in the periphery, especially in fat cells and skin, accounting for most of the circulating estrogen in postmenopausal women. This transitional phase, during which a woman passes out of the reproductive stage, begins before menopause. It is termed the climacteric or perimenopause, although many persons refer to it as menopause.

There are two obvious qualities to this text. First, all these biological processes are described in terms of decay and decline: ovaries age, hormone production decreases, and follicles fail; this language of decline as applied to female reproductive physiology has been characterized extremely well by Emily Martin (Martin 1992). Second, except for the first sentence of the description of symptoms (which range from "nonexistent to severe") it is phrased in a strictly absolutist language; given the "cause and effect" style of the analysis, it is hard to understand how some women might not have any symptoms. Note that whether or not they have symptoms, they are certainly said to "have" menopause. Indeed the *Manual* tells us under the heading of "Diagnosis" that "Menopause is usually obvious."

One imagines that such biological activity would be quite universal. Since everyone ages, and since ovarian function always more or less ceases, these symptoms would be expected to occur everywhere. But this doesn't seem to be the case. Margaret Lock has shown that menopause as a medical condition generally doesn't exist in Japan. In a detailed survey comparing several thousand older women in Japan, Manitoba, and Massachusetts, only 10% of Japanese women reported hot flashes in the previous two weeks, while they were reported by 31% and 35% of women in Manitoba and Massachusetts, respectively. Only 4% of Japanese women reported night sweats as opposed to 20% in Manitoba and 12% in Massachusetts. Lock writes "Movement through the life cycle is subjectively experienced [by Japanese] largely in terms of how one's relationships with other people shift through time, and for women particularly, life is expected to become meaningful according to what they accomplish for others rather than for themselves. . . . Under these circumstances the end of menstruation is not a very potent icon." And indeed, "there is . . . no widely used specific term in contemporary Japanese that expresses in everyday language the event of the end of menstruation" (Lock 1993; see also Lock 1986a). Lock notes elsewhere that "among Mayan Indians, North Africans resident in Israel, the Rajput of India, and Japanese the occurrence of somatic symptoms [associated with menopause] is reported to be either low or absent, [and while it has been shown that] the prevalence of hot flashes among Navajo and 'Anglos' are similar, their frequency is very different (while 65% to 70% of an Anglo sample reported experiencing hot flashes each day, only 17% of a Navajo sample reported them with that frequency). In contrast, studies in North America, Europe, ... Zimbabwe, ... and Varanasi, India elicit much higher symptom reporting" (Lock 1986b:7).

In so far as people (outside of medical anthropology) recognize variations like this at all they tend to explain them by recourse to some sort of racial theory, usually a theory of moral hierarchy. "We" – that is, white European-descended people, usually male – are "normal," and even quite wonderful. Others are somehow deviant, underdeveloped, or in decay.

The best example of this may be the long interest in anthropology in what were called "culture-bound syndromes" (see, for example Lebra 1976; Simons and Hughes 1985). Most of these – *amok, susto, latah*, and the like – were understood to be specific and culturally shaped illnesses of "other people." So, "we" had "biology" and "diseases," but "they" had "superstition" and "culture-bound syndromes." More recently, scholars have recognized that *all* illnesses are shaped and formed by meaning, by culture (Kleinman 1988).

I am uncertain of how biologists might respond to Lock's account of the absence of menopause among Japanese, Maya, and Rajput, but one imagines it will be a racialist explanation; that is, the Japanese or Maya will be seen to be a "different kind" of people, rather than people living a different kind of life, experiencing their bodies in different ways. This clearly is an inadequate and inappropriate way to understand the situation, as we can see in the following case.

An epidemic of ADHD

The United States is experiencing an incredible epidemic of Attention Deficit Hyperactivity Disorder (ADHD), one unknown in our own past or elsewhere in the world. Various estimates suggest that the number of children being treated with stimulants (typically methylphenidate or Ritalin) increased dramatically in the 1990s. One study showed a 2.5-fold increase in treatment of children between 1990 and 1995, and estimated that "2.8% (or 1.5 million) of US youths aged 5 to 18 were receiving this medication in mid-1995" (Safer, Zito, and Fine 1996). Another showed a three-fold increase in treatment of *preschool* children two to four years old from 1991 to 1995 (Zito *et al.* 2000). This is a particularly interesting case, and it shows how ordinary variations in human physiology can be made into "diseases" as cultural conditions change. A number of surveys around the world show that if one screens thousands of children, and applies to them strict observational criteria, varying numbers of "hyperactive" or "hyper kinetic" children can be identified, usually fewer than in the United States.[26] But nowhere is it *treated* with anywhere near the intensity that it is treated in the US. That is, in most places, it is not seen to be abnormal (except perhaps by the researchers). Why? The diagnosis of the condition is based on a checklist of symptoms in the DSM-IV[27] which includes statements like these: the child must display "inattention" by failing to "give close attention to details", or the child "makes careless mistakes in schoolwork," or "fails to finish schoolwork" or "often loses things necessary for tasks or activities (e.g., school assignments, pencils, books, tools, or toys)." Also, the child "often avoids or strongly dislikes . . . schoolwork or homework" and "often fidgets with hands or feet or squirms in seat." Of course, you can't have any of these symptoms if you don't have schools, and want them to be extremely quiet and orderly, with children confined to chairs. There is evidence to indicate that many American schools have eliminated recess, periods of unstructured play; schools have been built without any playgrounds. "We are intent on improving academic performance," said one big city school superintendent. "You don't do that by having kids hanging on the monkey bars" (Johnson 1999).

I recently asked my aunt about ADHD. She taught elementary school in an inner-city environment for ten years in the 1930s and again for ten years in the 1950s. I asked her if she had many students with ADHD. She said, "Well, there was Robert. We didn't know about ADHD then, but I have wondered if he might have had it." One can easily predict that 5% to 10% of the boys in the schools where my aunt taught are currently being given Ritalin every day. Changing expectations for proper behavior and for "school performance" are probably the major factors accounting for

---

[26] For Italy, see (Gallucci *et al.* 1993), for Israel, see (Zohar *et al.* 1992), for Hong Kong, see (Leung *et al.* 1996), for Iceland, see (Magnusson *et al.* 1999), for Colombia, see (Brewis, Schmidt, and Meyer 2000).

[27] The DSM-IV, or *Diagnostic and Statistical Manual of Mental Disorders*, published by the American Psychiatric Association, is a classification of mental illnesses (American Psychiatric Association 1994). There are other such classifications like the International Classification of Diseases (currently the tenth edition: ICD-10) which has a somewhat more restrictive definition of ADHD or what it terms "hyperkinetic disorder"; as a result, there are fewer hyperkinetic than hyperactive children.

this increase in ADHD. The extension of these expectations to preschool children is particularly interesting (and disturbing).

People characterize different things as "good to eat" and eat accordingly in different places. People in different places experience the same biological phenomena (cessation of menses, for example) extremely differently, to the point that in one place it is a disease, a condition to be treated with hormone replacement therapy, while in another place it is barely noticed. And, in the same culture, over a short period of time, behaviors which have existed for all time can be newly defined as diseases when they never were before, as with ADHD. These matters are not simply biological, but they involve some interaction of biology (digestion, ovarian function, activity or attention) with expectations, understandings, and meanings about those biological phenomena.

France, Germany, Britain, and the United States

In a fascinating and insightful book, Lynn Payer has characterized many different understandings of health, illness, sickness and treatment in the United States, Great Britain, France and Germany by both ordinary people and medical scientists, expanding broadly on an insight like Lock's on menopause (Payer 1996). In France, people routinely are diagnosed with conditions like *spasmophile, colibaccilose, crise de foie* (a "liver crisis"), and *fatigue*, conditions which simply don't exist elsewhere in the world. These things evolve: while "liver diseases" declined by a factor of four in the 1970s, in the same period spasmophile increased sevenfold.

Germans, by contrast, routinely diagnose a condition known as *Herzinsuffizienz*, a condition not recognized in France or the US (discussed in more detail later in this chapter). In severe forms, the German disease may be more or less the same as what American doctors call "congestive heart failure." But in its ordinary form, where its symptoms might include tiredness, urination at night, or edema of tissues (fluid accumulation in the limbs) – or with no symptoms at all – it is simply not diagnosed elsewhere; in Germany, it is treated with digitalis. German doctors prescribe digitalis (and related drugs) seven times as often as do French or British doctors. In the US, with a very aggressive medical culture, many things are treated which are not elsewhere: radical mastectomy is still very common, although it practically doesn't occur elsewhere; very modestly elevated blood pressure is treated widely in the US; and while there may not be much spasmophile, there is an abundance of "virus" or "low-grade virus" infection which doesn't appear in the experience of other people in the world.

These different diseases, then, are very common. Even among advanced technological societies sharing a rich scientific tradition, very different understandings of and experiences of biology can occur. These different interpretations of biology can have very profound effects on people; they can have significant impact on life and death, on mortality itself.

Chinese astrology

A large study – very methodologically sophisticated – examined the cause of death of 28,169 adult Chinese-Americans and nearly half a million randomly selected matched "white" controls, all from California. It was found that "Chinese-Americans, but not whites, die significantly earlier than normal (1.3–4.9 yr) if they have a combination of disease and birth year which Chinese astrology and medicine consider ill fated" (Phillips *et al.* 1993:1142). For example, among the Chinese-Americans whose deaths were attributed to lymphatic cancer (n = 3,041), those who were born in "Earth years" – and consequently were deemed, by Chinese medical theory, especially susceptible to diseases involving lumps, nodules, or tumors – had an average age at death (AAD) of 59.7 years; among those born in other years, AAD of Chinese-Americans also suffering from lymphatic cancer was 63.6 years, nearly four years longer. Similarly, for Chinese-Americans who died of illnesses related to lung diseases (bronchitis, emphysema and asthma), those who were born in "Metal years" – "the Lung [is] the organ of Metal" (Beinfield and Korngold 1991:204) – had an average AAD of 66.9 years; among those born in other years, AAD of those dying from such lung diseases was 71.9 years, five years longer. Similar differences were found for other sorts of cancers, for heart attack, and for a series of other diseases. No such differences were evident in a large series of "whites" who died of similar causes in the same period. The intensity of the effect was shown to be correlated with "the strength of commitment to traditional Chinese culture." It is clear from this case that these significant differences in longevity among Chinese-Americans (up to 6 or 7 percent of length of life!) is not due to having Chinese genes, but to having Chinese ideas, to knowing the world in Chinese ways.

Shots and pills again

In Chapter 5, I summarized a meta-analysis which had shown that injected placebo worked better for migraine than oral placebo, and suggested that this was a consequence of the different meanings of injections

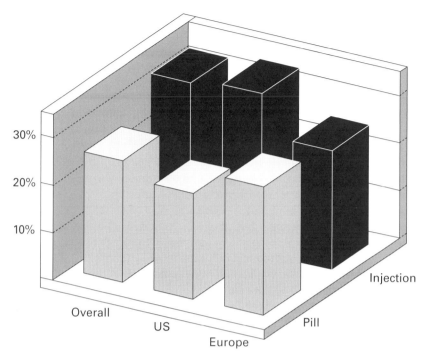

6.1 Inert injections are more effective for migraine in the United States, but not in Europe (*Source*: de Craen *et al.* 2000)

and pills. There is, however, more to the study than that. Overall, in twenty-two studies, the relief rate for oral placebo was 25.7% while the relief rate for injected placebo was 32.4% (6.7% difference). Shots work better than pills.

In studies which were carried out in the United States, the same pattern appeared: 22.3% oral vs. 33.6% subcutaneous placebo relief rate. In studies done in Europe however, the difference disappeared: 27.1% oral vs. 25.1% subcutaneous placebo relief rate (see Figure 6.1) (de Craen *et al.* 2000:186). Shots work better than pills, but only in the US. There are cultural differences shaping the placebo effect.

This shows up another way. Only 20% of American patients received oral placebo, while 80% got shots. In Europe, 68% got oral treatments while only 32% got shots. Americans "know" that shots work better than pills and so, they give shots. Europeans are apparently less certain about these matters. The knowledge and understanding that people have about medicine makes a difference in how effective it is, and in how medicine is practiced.

Ulcer treatment here and there

There are other examples of this sort of cross-cultural variation. In the late 1970s, a wonderful new drug appeared on the scene called cimetidine, sold in the United States under the name Tagamet. It was the first really effective drug for healing ulcers. In 1977, a group of researchers in France did a randomized controlled trial of cimetidine. They gathered a large number of patients with the symptoms of ulcers and examined them with an endoscope, the fiber optic device which allowed them to look at the inside of the stomach. They found 140 people with ulcers of the duodenum who agreed to join the trial of the new drug. They were randomly assigned to receive the new drug or a matching placebo. They each took a 200 mg tablet after each meal, and two tablets at bed time for a total of 1,000 mg. After four weeks, they were checked again with the endoscope, and then the study was "unblinded." It turned out that 54 of the 71 patients who took cimetidine were better (76%), as were 41 of 69 patients who took placebo (59%) (Lambert *et al.* 1977). Although this was a statistically significant difference, it doesn't look like a very significant practical difference; the difference between the two groups is only 17%, and nearly 6 of 10 patients were better after a month taking inert medication!

Shortly after, another group of researchers in Brazil did a similar study. They, too, found a group of people with duodenal ulcers using the endoscope and randomly divided them into two groups. They took pills four times a day, one at each meal, and two at bedtime; one group took 200 mg tablets of cimetidine, and the other group took inert placebos. After four weeks, 15 of 25 patients taking cimetidine were better (60%), and 3 of the 29 who took placebos were better (10%) (Salgado *et al.* 1981). This, too, was a statistically significant difference, but it's a big difference this time.

There is quite a difference, too, between the results of these two studies. In France, three-quarters of the drug patients got better, while in Brazil 60% got better. The bigger difference is in the placebo-treated patients: in France 60% of them got better, while in Brazil only 10% got better. It is worth noting that the same proportion of French patients treated with *placebo* got better (59%) as did Brazilian patients treated with *cimetidine* (60%).

I first noticed these substantial variations in the placebo effect about twenty years ago, and have kept track of them ever since. The situation is somewhat complicated (as is appropriate for human beings!) and very interesting.

Consider the case of Germany. Among 117 trials I have found of drugs for treating ulcers, the placebo healing rate in six studies in Germany averages 59%, twice as high as in the rest of the world (statistically significant; there is one chance in 10,000 that this is a random result) and three times that of two of its neighboring countries, Denmark and the Netherlands, where, in five studies, it averages 22% (one chance in a hundred). Given the available evidence, the placebo healing rate for ulcers in Germany is much higher than in the rest of the world. Why is this so?

I do not know. Colleagues and students, when told of the German data on ulcers, often break into their best "Hogan's Heroes" accent and assert that German doctors must tell their patients that "You vill get better!" The notion that medicine is somehow more authoritarian in Germany than elsewhere is not, however, borne out by others who know more about the situation. German medicine is probably the most holistic of any Western European country and shows a strong concern with emotional balance; regular spa treatment is still routinely covered by the national health care system (Maretzki 1987; Payer 1996). Germany is well known for widespread use of herbal medicines and a broad range of constitutional cures.

To look more closely, I expanded the study beyond ulcers and examined more than 400 studies of drugs for the treatment of moderate high blood pressure or hypertension from around the world; thirty-two studies provided data which allowed me to compare them to one another. Overall, active drug treatment reduced diastolic blood pressure (DBP; the "small number" in blood pressure) by an average of 10.9 mm of mercury ("Hg"; the range was from 7 to 21), while placebo treatment reduced DBP by 3.5 mm Hg (range –5 to 9; in two studies, placebo-treated patients had an increase in mean DBP). Systolic blood pressure (SBP; the big number) was reduced on average by 15.9 mm Hg (range 7 to 28), while placebo treatment reduced SBP by 3.9 mm Hg (range –6 to 15).

In this broad range of studies two things were obvious. First, blood pressure could be reduced by taking active medication, but it could also be reduced by taking inert drugs, placebos. What about Germany? The mean placebo group change in DBP in four German trials was only .25 mm Hg, while in the remaining twenty-nine trials it was 3.9 (chance occurrence one time in 66). One of the German studies showed an *increase* of 5 mm Hg in DBP with placebo treatment. The placebo effect for lowering blood pressure in Germany is the lowest of any place represented in the thirty-two studies.

What this suggests is that, at least for Germany, the high or low placebo effect is not a generalized phenomenon, but specific to different diseases. It may be possible in this case to suggest something of what is going on. For example, German medicine and culture have an unusually strong concern with the "heart" and its workings; I put the word in quotation marks to indicate that I am describing ideas that people have about the "heart," not the heart itself. Payer (1996) notes that Germans, but not French, British, or Americans, regularly diagnose and treat low blood pressure; in the United States, such treatment in otherwise normal individuals would probably be considered malpractice. She also notes that even though the Germans have nearly the same rate of heart disease as do the French and English, they use *six times* the amount of heart medication as their neighbors do. When reading electrocardiograms, German doctors find that roughly 40% of patients need some sort of treatment; using American criteria to read the same tests, about 5% would get some treatment. One doctor told Payer that "any patient who was about sixty years old and had any one of three symptoms – extreme tiredness, urination at night or edema (water logging of tissues) – suffered from *Herzinsuffizienz* and should be given digitalis to prevent further deterioration" (Payer 1996:82).

This uncommon German view of blood pressure may be related to the low placebo effect in the treatment of *high* blood pressure there; concern about their blood pressure getting too low may inhibit their response to antihypertensive treatment. Or it may not. But it seems clear that, in different Western nations, people have very different ideas about the "same" medical conditions (actually, given these different ideas, the conditions aren't the "same" any more). Such differences in the ways people live in their bodies can clearly make a difference in the way they react to illness, treatment, and medication.

I don't have a similar story for Brazil where, in three studies, the average placebo healing rate for ulcers is 7% compared to 36% in the rest of the world (chance difference one time in 625). When I have explained this to Brazilian colleagues they have told me simply that I was wrong, that it couldn't be true. I don't know why it couldn't, and I have no idea why, say, Germans and Brazilians are so different on this score. It is important to note, as we have before, that these are not simply "placebo effects." The difference between Germans and Brazilians on placebo effects (in the strict sense) for ulcer treatment (59% vs. 7%) is a statistically significant one (it could be a chance occurrence once in 100 times). But it is also the case that there is a big difference between the drug healing rates for ulcers in these two places. The German rate is 78% and the Brazilian is 54%; this could be a chance occurrence one time in 32. That is, the variation in the placebo effectiveness rate carries over to the drug healing rate – the correlation between the two for all 117 studies is 0.4; for 55 more similar cases of duodenal ulcers treated with cimetidine, the correlation is 0.53. Whatever is going on is not confined to people taking inert medication, but applies to all people.

Conclusions

In different parts of the world, people define different things as edible, and, therefore, eat different things. In different parts of the world, people might eat the same things, but they may organize their cuisine differently enough that an outsider eating it – eating familiar foods in unfamiliar ways – might find that the food was not satisfying, it didn't give a feeling of having eaten. Acupuncture is more effective when it is experienced than when it is hidden; similarly, pain medication is more effective when you know you are getting it from a clinician than when it is administered secretly.

Menopause and ADHD vary dramatically in their occurrence in different cultures even though the physiology (of the ovaries) or the behavior (inattention, activity) seem to be more or less the same the world around: In China and Colombia as well as the US, many young boys have a hard time sitting still in school. In the US, but not Colombia, this is a "disorder" treated with Ritalin. Chinese-Americans, but not the neighboring Anglo-Americans down the street, know that certain birth years are auspicious (or not) regarding certain diseases, and it has a significant effect on their life spans.

Injections of saline solution are more effective than inert pills in the United States, but not in Europe. And there are dramatic differences in the effectiveness of inert pills in the treatment of ulcer disease around the world.

The things that we "know" in our different cultures around the world, and which vitalize our lives, vary dramatically, whether it is what we know to be the proper meal, appropriate dress, the correct behavior for older women, or good behavior in school (assuming there *are* schools). The same is true for the illnesses from which we suffer that, even under the conditions of a widely shared conventional scientific medicine, vary significantly, and have different portents and meanings in different places. In such a world, where meaning shapes so much of life, it is not surprising that meaning also influences the effectiveness of medical treatment.

There is more to biology than biology. This isn't always the case (leaping from a sixteenth-story window ledge will not be much affected by desire, will, or culture). But far more often than we realize, what appears to be an "obvious" biological matter is richly freighted with meaning, history, tradition, or the like; or requires consciousness to do its thing. Indeed, it is probably wise to assume this is the case until it's proven otherwise.

We have seen in these cases that there is good reason to believe that different beliefs in different parts of the world can have substantial effects on human biology. These issues raise some fascinating problems. The preponderance of American readers, while being polite, will not share the Chinese view that people born in earth years will have more difficulty with lung diseases than people born in other years; indeed, Anglo-Californians did not show the same pattern of mortality that was seen among Chinese-Americans. Similarly, one could imagine that Europeans might maintain a healthy skepticism toward the American preference for injections rather than pills; and, indeed, placebo injections work better in America than in Europe. What is true in one community seems not to be true in another. What, then, *is* true?

One scholar who has thought about this is James Dow, who has written widely on medicine among non-Western peoples, especially the Otomi Indians of Mexico. Dow tells us that, if an Otomi feels troubled or confused about something happening in his life, he might approach a shaman. The Otomi word for shaman is *vǫdi* which is derived from the word *pǫdi* which means "to know." Shamans have visions through which they gain knowledge. "Knowledge," Dow writes, "is not just belief; it is something that is true for many people" (Dow 1986a:49). Elsewhere, addressing the same issue, he differentiates between two different sorts of knowledge, "experiential knowledge" and "empirical knowledge." Any human world, he says, "contains knowledge that is experientially, but not necessarily empirically, true" (Dow 1986b). It is, however, more paradoxical even than this. The experiential knowledge of the Chinese-Americans regarding birth years seems to be empirically true for them, but not for Anglo-Americans. The experiential knowledge of Americans regarding injections seems to be empirically true for them, but not for Europeans. Although not quite so clear, it seems plausible to suggest that whatever is experientially true about ulcer disease for Germans has a quite different empirical consequence for them than whatever is experientially true for the Brazilians.

In so far as a culture (German, Navajo, Zulu) is a skein of meanings, understandings, beliefs, and knowledge, stitched together somehow by metaphors, institutions, and memories, and in so far as these things can affect individual lives, it seems reasonable to anticipate that these factors will work themselves out differently in different places in the world, even places as similar as Germany and Holland, Britain and the USA. The same item (a cimetidine tablet, or a placebo cimetidine tablet) can be expected to mean different things in such different places, and, therefore, it can be expected to have different effects there.

Part II

Applications, challenges, and opportunities

7 Psychotherapy: placebo effect or meaning response?

In the next two chapters, I will look closely at two areas where meaning is particularly effective: psychotherapy and physical pain.

Everyone has won and all must have prizes

Psychotherapy is a complex and contested business. Few doubt its effects, but many (at least many outside the field) are unsure of how to think about its effectiveness. Indeed, some have argued that psychotherapy is "only" the placebo effect. I will argue that this is good reason both to stop using the concept of the placebo effect in such a way, and to start thinking about the meaning response.

How does psychotherapy work? The simple answer is, "No one knows" (Dawes 1994:61–2). This is quite surprising and seems at variance with experience. Anyone who has ever peeked behind the surface of any sort of psychotherapy knows that practitioners have very strong views of how and why their practice works. Don't psychoanalysts know how their therapy works? Surely the behaviorists know what they are about and how things work. Of course they do, in some sense. But the problem is that both of these systems work, they seem to work more or less equally well, and they work equally well for the same sorts of problems.

There are huge differences in the attitudes, approaches, and theories underlying the different therapeutic schools – Freudian psychoanalysis and Skinnerian behavior therapy are about as different as one might imagine two approaches could possibly be when addressing, say, compulsive hand washing. There are literally dozens, perhaps hundreds, of such different "schools": Psychoanalytic, Adlerian, Eclectic, Transactional, Rational-emotive, Gestalt, Client-centered (Rogerian), Behaviorist approaches, etc., etc. Most of these can be short-term or long-term treatments, and aimed at individuals, groups, or families; and psychotherapists can be trained as physicians, as psychologists, as social workers, and a variety of other things. One authority has counted 418 different forms (he calls them "brand names"!) of therapy (Parloff 1986). Each of these cross-tabulations yields a group of practitioners who, typically, defend their approach as the "correct" one, better than the others. Psychotherapy, to an outsider, is reminiscent of Protestantism, where only fairly close study allows you to detect the differences between Presbyterians, Baptists, and Methodists; yet the adherents of each faith are clear in their identities.

The remarkable thing is that there is quite convincing evidence that all of these forms of psychotherapy are effective, and *they are all equally effective*! There have been several major studies comparing the effectiveness of different sorts of psychotherapy and, although they differ in their methods, they come to much the same conclusion. Probably the most widely known of these studies is one by Lester Luborsky and his colleagues titled "Comparative Studies of Psychotherapies: Is It True That 'Everyone Has Won and All Must Have Prizes?' "[28] After reviewing about forty different studies, the article concluded, yes, all have won: "For comparisons of [different sorts of] psychotherapy with each other, most studies found insignificant differences in proportions of patients who improved (though most patients benefitted)" (Luborsky, Singer, and Luborsky 1975). They also note that "even a fair proportion of patients who go through minimal treatment seem to make some gains. . . . This," they add, "may have contributed to our surprising finding that approximately a third of comparisons of psychotherapy with control groups do not show significant differences." In most of these cases, the control group is made up of a similar group of people with similar complaints who are evaluated, and then simply placed on a waiting list, given "minimal psychotherapy" – one short session discussing problems with a therapist – or hospital care alone. While 20 of 33 (61%) such studies showed that psychotherapy was better than the control, in 13 studies (39%), the outcome was more or less a tie (in none of the studies did the control group do better than the treatment group). But the important thing is that even in those studies where it was a tie, most of the patients got better!

As you might imagine, this was a very controversial study; it is rather as if some heavenly researcher managed to determine that most Protestants went to heaven, and the proportions saved were not different for the Baptists, the Presbyterians, the Methodists, or the Quakers. Not surprisingly, other studies followed.

A massive comparison of 375 studies of different sorts of psychotherapy, using quite different (and quite sophisticated) statistical methods came to much the same conclusions, and provided "convincing evidence of the efficacy of psychotherapy. On the average, the typical therapy client

---

[28] The quotation comes from Lewis Carroll's *Alice in Wonderland*, while the dodo bird serves as the judge in a race.

is better off than 75% of untreated individuals" (Smith and Glass 1977). And, as Luborsky found, "Despite volumes devoted to the theoretical differences among different schools of psychotherapy, the results of research demonstrate negligible differences in the effects produced by different therapy types" (Smith and Glass 1977:760).

It is not clear to me what the predispositions of these investigators were; whether, for example, they hoped to find more or less what they did. Smith and Glass seem to be rather hostile towards behavior therapies, and seem to attempt to show that they are no more effective than psychodynamic therapies; their data appear to me to show that the behaviorists have a slight edge (a very slight one, to be sure), but it seems to me that they attempt to minimize it. In this context, the study by Landman and Dawes is rather different (Landman and Dawes 1982). Dawes quite explicitly attests that he was sceptical of the findings of Smith and Glass, and doubted that psychotherapy was as effective as they said it was (Dawes 1994:52). In particular, they thought that many of the studies Smith and Glass used did not really have random allocation to the different groups; this could make a big difference. So they went through the 375 studies (plus an additional 60 they added), and selected out only those which seemed to have genuinely random allocation of patients to the various study groups. They added a few additional criteria to be certain they had only the highest quality studies; then they selected every fifth study for close analysis, for a total sample of 65. Of these, they concluded that only 42 had used true random assignment of patients to the different treatment groups. Using the same methods as Smith and Glass, they compared the 42 studies to the 65, and found that "much to our surprise, our results were virtually identical to those of Smith and Glass. That is, it didn't matter whether the studies had had true random assignment." Dawes reported that he had become a "reformed sinner" – he had originally believed that much of the apparent success of psychotherapy was due to faulty research methodology, but now he was a "true believer"; psychotherapy was very effective regardless of its theories (Dawes 1994:54).

The professional reaction to these studies was quite mixed. On the one hand, everyone was quite happy that psychotherapy could be shown to help so many people. On the other hand, no one could use the studies to say "my kind of therapy is best"; quite the contrary, the best that anyone could say is "any form of therapy is as good as any other." And there was another finding, most clearly shown in the study by Smith and Glass. Curiously enough, even though it is perfectly obvious in one of their tables, they never actually mention in their text that there is no relationship at all between the effectiveness of any form of psychotherapy and the amount of experience of the therapist. One fairly common critique of studies of psychotherapy is that experienced therapists are often unwilling to participate in such studies; they know how to treat their patients, and they are often unwilling to work with patients according to some other sort of theory. As a result, the therapists in many studies of psychotherapy are medical students or residents who have to do more or less what they are told, and who don't have much experience. So Smith and Glass were careful to note how much experience the therapists had. The correlation of effect size (the measure of effectiveness of the particular form of psychotherapy) with the experience of the psychotherapist was -0.01 – that is, effectively zero.

This finding has been replicated on several occasions: there is little evidence to indicate that the most experienced, educated, and credentialed (and expensive) psychotherapists are any more effective in their treatment of patients than are stripling social workers still in training. It is very important to remember that this does not say that psychotherapy is not effective!! Rather, the most and the least experienced therapists have substantial (and more or less equal) effectiveness.

Professors as therapists

Perhaps the best demonstration of this is seen in a study by Strupp and Hadley, who identified a series of disturbed college students and allocated half of them to practicing psychotherapists (averaging twenty-three years of experience). The other half were allocated to a group of college professors of English, philosophy, history or mathematics, people who were selected on the basis of their "reputation for warmth, trustworthiness, and interest in students," and were of the same general age and professional status as the therapists, but had no previous experience as therapists. There were two other groups of students established as controls, one which received minimal treatment and one which was only given diagnostic testing. Over a period of a year, all the groups showed mean improvements in most measures. In part, this study shows the power of "regression to the mean," which was discussed in Chapter 3; under some circumstances, people selected on the basis of being extreme on one or another diagnostic test often improve over some period of time. However, the students who received up to twenty-five hours of discussion with either the therapists or the professors did significantly better than the control groups. But there were no significant differences between the improvement of those who spoke with the therapists or with the professors. There was a significant amount of variation within each group, which led to some interesting observations. "Our results suggest that the positive changes experienced by our patients, whether they were treated by a [therapist] or a [professor], are generally attributable to the healing effects of a benign human relationship. More specifically, therapeutic change seemed to occur when there was a conjunction between a patient who was capable of taking advantage of such a relationship (i.e., not too resistant and highly motivated) and a therapist whose interventions were experienced by the patient as expressions of caring and genuine interest" (Strupp and Hadley 1979).

One counter-example, which suggests that certain types of pairing of patient and psychiatrist (what the authors call "matchmaking") work better than others, indicates something of the complexity of the situation: "The results indicate that interactions between patient and therapist self-concept were associated with outcome. More specifically, this occurred when the affiliation dimension of the circumplex was used as the independent variable" (Talley, Strupp, and Morey 1990). Unfortunately, I have no idea what this means. It's hard to imagine how one might, in a practical manner, use this information as a guide to selecting the best psychiatrist for your own situation. The best conclusion for the moment is that one is as good as another.

So, how does psychotherapy work? Placebo or meaning?

Since the 1960s, the most thoughtful approach to this issue has been Jerome Frank's. Frank, a psychotherapist who spent most of his career at Johns Hopkins, is probably best known today for a fascinating book titled *Persuasion and Healing* originally published in 1961. In it, he proposed the then-radical notion that all forms of psychotherapy, as different as they were on the surface, worked because they contained similar elements: a helping relationship with a thoughtful listener, a clearly defined healing space, and a "ritual" of some sort to cement the relationship between the healer and the patient. He also argued that there was really only one underlying psychological illness, which he called "demoralization." He meant this, I believe, in the metaphorical sense of the term – to be demoralized was to have had one's power of bearing up against dangers, fatigue or difficulties damaged, to have lost one's "morale," or spirit. Frank, a man in his prime during the Second World War and the Cold War, wrote widely of the destructive psychological effect on people of living in fear of nuclear war. And he noted that these elements were common to psychological healing across time and space, and in a broad range of cultures in non-Western and primitive societies. He said, too, that these factors were "non-specific." In that, he meant that they occurred in all therapeutic systems. (He may not have actually looked at 418 different systems, but he is certainly right that these factors occur in all the significant ones!)

In the past, attacks against such a formulation have had a particular character and have accused psychotherapy of having *no* effect. The best known such attack is probably that of Dr. Hans Eysenck, who argued that all the changes attributed to psychotherapy were in fact due to "spontaneous remission," or what today might be termed "regression to the mean" (Eysenck 1952; Eysenck 1994). There clearly is such change in certain psychiatric problems, but it seems extremely unlikely that it accounts for all of the improvement people experience.

A more challenging attack is described this way by one researcher: "The invective *placebo* has recently been invoked with increasing shrillness to account for the positive effects of psychotherapy" (Parloff 1986; see also Laporte and Figueras 1994). Why is it an "invective?" I am reminded of the two acupuncturists I described earlier who accused one another of using techniques which were "only placebo." And if a placebo is something which is inert, and which has no effect, then psychotherapy has a bit of a problem.

To say that psychotherapy is simply a placebo effect sounds like invective, indeed. To me, it sounds much more reasonable to say that psychotherapy evokes meaning responses. A generation ago, the great anthropologist Claude Levi-Strauss compared the techniques of the shaman and the psychoanalyst; he began by analyzing a long myth of the Cuna Indians of Panama, a myth which is utilized to facilitate difficult childbirth. "In both [the shamanic and the psychoanalytic] cases the purpose is to bring to a conscious level conflicts and resistance which have remained unconscious ... The shamanistic cure seems to be the exact counterpart to the psychoanalytic cure, but with an inversion of all the elements. Both cures aim at inducing an experience, and both succeed by recreating a myth which the patient has to live or relive. But in one case, the patient constructs an individual myth with elements drawn from his past; in the other case, the patient receives from the outside a social myth which does not correspond to a former personal state" (Levi-Strauss 1967a:193–4). In Levi-Strauss' view, the patient, the shaman or psychoanalyst, and the community, come together in various ways to create a myth, a construct of meaning, from some elements of distress. He, like Frank, sees the common elements surrounding helping relationships, context, and ritual. But he sees them as subordinate to the meanings constructed in such a way that "the cure would consist, therefore, in making explicit a situation originally existing on the emotional level and in rendering acceptable to the mind pains [in this case of childbirth] which the body refuses to tolerate ... [And more generally,] the effectiveness of symbols would consist precisely in this 'inductive property,' by which formally homologous structures, built out of different materials at different levels of life – organic processes, unconscious mind, rational thought – are related to one another" (*ibid.*: 192, 197).

In Levi-Strauss' view, the processes are the same, but that's subordinate to the crystallization of experience into meaningful symbols, particularly metaphors, which can, he says citing Rimbaud, "change the world."

In what is certainly a less colorful, and more bounded, argument, Strupp (who designed the therapist/professor study), rather as Levi-Strauss suggests, provides an analogous account, but with an "inversion of the elements." He focuses on the psychotherapeutic "process" and says it contains four elements. First, therapists are guided by a theory. This, he says, provides therapists with a kind of intensity, with a depth of purpose which can keep them engaged for the long term. He notes that the college professors in the comparative project, who had no such theory to fall back on, tended to "run out of material" and were "at a loss to explain how one patient's 'girl trouble' might be improved by further conversations." Second, the therapist creates and maintains "a particular *interpersonal context*," characterized by "empathic listening." Third, through this careful contextual listening, "the therapist seeks to *understand the meaning* of the patient's feelings, wishes, fantasies, beliefs, action patterns, etc." Fourth, the therapist attempts to "reformulate ('interpret')" these meanings as they have emerged "with certain affective charge ... in a way that the patient can productively assimilate" them (Strupp 1986).

Of course, Dr. Strupp is interested more in the problem of how therapists heal than in how people get better. Look again at his four points from the *patient's* point of view. The very fact that the therapist has a *theory* of human difficulty encourages the patient to recognize the possibility that whatever it is that's bothering him may have happened before, to someone else. This is a powerful idea for someone suffering mightily with serious depression, or is experiencing a divorce, or the loss of a loved one, or similar emotional pain. This guy, who seems to know about such things, doesn't appear to be in nearly as much agony as I am. Second, a therapist can only be an empathic listener if the patient is willing to talk; and, of course, after you have told your "girl trouble" to your roommate, or your mother, for the third or fourth time, they don't want to hear it again. But it still hurts, it still nags and enrages and frustrates you. For people who are depressed, it is often incredibly difficult to talk about it at all with anyone (your sister says "Cheer up" and your mother cries); here is someone who knows how to talk about depression. And the guy keeps listening. Maybe by the sixth or eighth time you say it, it won't hurt so much any more. Third, he takes it seriously – he seems to think that my unhappiness *means* something; and not only that, but (fourth), even though I have been crying like a baby [that's what Dr. Strupp called a "certain affective charge"], he's willing to take it seriously, and interpret it with me. We work out an understanding for me (a myth, in Levi-Strauss' terms) which makes sense of the inchoate, the anomalous, the unapproachable. "The vocabulary matters less than the structure. Whether the myth is re-created by the individual or borrowed from the tradition, it derives from its sources – individual or collective (between which interpenetrations and exchanges constantly occur) – only the stock of representations with which it operates. But the structure remains the same, and through it the symbolic function is fulfilled" (Levi-Strauss 1967a:199).

In an interview in 1998, Jerome Frank put it this way: "Psychotherapy is not applied behavior science. I think that is the wrong model. Because all science is based on facts, but psychotherapy is the world of meanings, which is far from the world of facts. Psychotherapy relies on the fact that human beings react not to the facts or events themselves *but to the meanings of the facts as they interpret them*. Psychotherapy is the transformation of the meanings that patients attribute to events from negative to positive. I think it should be taught as an art" (Holland and Guerra 1998).

This probably won't satisfy Dr. Eysenck. But it seems clear enough that the fact of talking about "demoralization" might "remoralize" me, might reshape my sense of who and what I am, and that this might relieve some of the pain of life, does *not* seem to me to be aptly described as a "placebo effect," but it does seem to be a powerful response to meaning which I have constructed with the help of a therapist. Psychotherapy is a rich example of the powers of the meaning response.

Meaning and disclosure

Another body of research leads to similar conclusions, but in a way that shows us how a little meaning can have a big impact. In the 1980s, James Pennebaker, a psychologist at the University of Texas, began a series of fascinating experiments, initially with college students in introductory psychology classes. The experiments varied in a number of ways, but the basic structure was usually something like this: the college students were told to write about an assigned topic for fifteen minutes a day for four days. They were randomly divided into two groups. One group, the control group, was told to write about everyday, ordinary phenomena – to describe the laboratory room where the experiment was taking place, or their own living room, or the like. The other group was told to write about their very deepest thoughts and feelings regarding the most traumatic experience of their lives. They were told to explore their deepest emotions and thoughts, to include their feelings about their relations with others, with their parents, friends, lovers – in a phrase, to let it all out. The researchers were astonished at the students' responses. First, they took immediately to the task, and wrote long and engaging stories, often telling of truly awful experiences in gripping and persuasive prose. The students also told the researchers that they had enjoyed these emotional moments (many cried while writing), and would readily do it again. They found it psychologically positive and helpful.

But the most striking result of this experiment lay elsewhere. For the rest of the school year, Pennebaker followed up on the students in his experiment, in particular checking to see how often they visited the university health center in the months after the experiment. He found that the students who had written about their thoughts and feelings went to the clinic far less often than did the students who had written about mundane things. Writing about traumatic events had not only a positive psychological effect, it also had a positive effect on the students' physical health.

This simple experiment has been repeated in dozens of settings in the past fifteen years or so; people have varied the experimental conditions one way or another. People have written more or less; the writings have been public or private; in some experiments, people were asked to talk (not write) about their traumas; the people writing have been senior corporate executives, or prison inmates, or medical students, distressed crime-victims, people with chronic pain, or men laid off from their jobs, among others. Such studies have been done in the US, New Zealand, the Netherlands, Belgium, and Mexico City. Almost always the results seem to be the same: there is a positive health effect of some sort. Many of these experiments have been described in Dr. Pennebaker's book *Opening Up* (Pennebaker 1990).

Here are a few examples. In one study, Holocaust survivors were asked to talk for an hour or two about their personal experiences during the Second World War; the talks were videotaped. The videotapes were analyzed in several ways to determine how traumatic the person's disclosure was, and the thirty-three people were rated on the total amount of traumatic material they had disclosed. About fourteen months after their interview, each person was contacted again and asked how their health had been during the past year. Controlling for the number of health problems people had before the interview, the "degree of disclosure during the interview was found to be positively correlated with long-term health after the interview" (Pennebaker, Barger, and Tiebout 1989).

In another study, medical students were randomly assigned to write about personal traumatic events or various control topics for four daily sessions. On the fifth day, they were given a vaccination for hepatitis B with boosters after one and four months. Blood was collected before each vaccination and at a six-month follow-up. "Compared with the control group, participants in the emotional expression group showed significantly higher antibody levels against hepatitis B at the 4- and 6-month follow up periods" (Petrie *et al.* 1995).

After such a disclosure, it appears that people go to the doctor less often, they report that they have had better health, and their immune systems seems to operate more effectively. The results have been quite dramatic especially since the "experimental condition" (write, or talk, about traumatic events for an hour or so) seems so minor. In more recent research, Pennebaker has tried to figure out why some trauma writers have more positive results than other. He has concluded, essentially, that they write better stories – stories which are more coherent, more persuasive, better organized. In a word, their stories seem (to me) to be more *meaningful*.

Moreover, he has found greater improvement in writers who, over the course of several writing sessions, changed their point of view. That is, if they started writing from a "private" perspective ("I thought such and such") to writing from a more inclusive perspective ("My wife and I believed that"), regardless of the "direction" of such change, they showed more health improvement than those who maintained one point of view, even if the story got better in the retelling. Transforming the story this way, telling the same story in a new way, from the point of view of different participants, or groups of participants, is, perhaps, a way in which people can create multiple meanings (what anthropologists technically call "polysemy"); the fact that there is a new perspective in the later story doesn't change the value of the perspective in the earlier one. But now there are two stories rather than only one. There is, perhaps, twice as much meaning and, thereby, more healing.

What happens when you tell someone a story about anguish and pain? You have to take a whole complex experience which you may have only partly understood at the time, and turn it into something coherent and understandable. In order to be understandable to someone else, the chances are it has to be understandable ("meaningful") to you. Many things that occur in our daily lives are, apparently, random (that is, not meaningful; they are just things that "happen"). Maybe, that particular event didn't just "happen" but maybe it has some "reason" (that is, it was meaningful – this thing that happened occurred because of some other thing which happened, and so the one thing is connected to, represents, implies, the other; the one thing "means" the other). How is one to tell which things that occur in a life are really happening to me for some reason, or are just the sort of random events of everyday life? I, of course, have no answer for this question in the abstract. Everyone answers it him-self (or doesn't, as the case may be). But to answer it is to detect, or to infer, or to find, meaning in events, and so to make events meaningful. John, at the age of 7, was on the playground with the little girl next door, Megan. A storm blew up; and before the rain came down, a huge bolt of lightning came out of the sky and hit the slide on which Megan was sliding. She was killed by the lightning. John had just urged Megan to go down the slide ("Nyah nyah! You can't go down the slide!!"). But it's never this simple. Andrew hadn't really wanted to play outside; he had wanted to watch television, or play video games, or figure out how to blow up his brother Jimmy with his chemistry set. But his mom said that it would be good for him to go outside and play with Megan, but that he should come back inside if it started raining. Obviously, I could go on here, adding detail after detail (the family had decided not to go to Cape Cod for the week because ..., etc.). How does Andrew ever tell this story to himself, or anyone else? What does he include, and what does he leave out? The results of Dr. Pennebaker's studies suggest that it doesn't make much difference what he leaves in and what he takes out. What is important is that he tells the story, that he puts in what he wants to and leaves out what he wants to, and that he *clarifies* for himself what the story is about. To do so is to make a significant improvement in his life, at least in so far as the experience was a traumatic one – note that "trauma" comes from the Greek word which means "injury," but the word is also somehow related to the notion of a "dream"; the German word for dream is "der Traum," and "to dream" is "träumen." Dreams are, perhaps, the single most "interpretable" things in our lives.

Conclusions

Psychotherapists help us create stories, "myths," which render our demoralization less painful, or, perhaps, "remoralize" us. But, as Dr. Pennebaker has shown, therapists are apparently not necessary for people to create their myths, to tell their stories. They probably help. But the story, the nexus of meaning, is what seems to heal.

Our stories are all unique; but they are never *only* unique. We never create our stories outside of place or time, outside of a cultural context of which we are often unaware. But it is clearly there, and it is the single biggest source of meaning in our lives.

8 The neurobiology and cultural biology of pain

Telling stories about our lives, or creating meaning from grief, can affect our bodies, our biology. Such meaning responses can occur within a broad range of medical or health phenomena: heart disease, ulcer disease, immune diseases, and so on. But the best-known biological system which displays impressive meaning responses is the body's pain system. This chapter will review the neurobiology and the cultural biology of the human pain system and show how meaning can influence the experience of pain.

Neurology of pain

Pain is an extremely important biological process, a powerful signal an organism uses to signal *to itself* that "something is wrong." To lack a sense of pain is to open yourself up to injury which, unrecognized, could easily be fatal. Pain is a primary device for learning. Unfortunately, the pain system can occasionally go awry, causing more trouble than it resolves. In this brief review we will touch only the high points, but you should gain some sense of the value, and the problems, of pain.

Some time ago, Dr. Alan Leslie summarized the case of a very sick man.

I am thinking of a sixty year old man with a cardiac aneurysm [a bulge in one of the walls of the heart] which developed following a coronary occlusion [heart attack]. After some years of auricular fibrillation [irregular heartbeat] and bare maintenance of compensation at absolute rest this man had an aortic saddle embolization [blockage of the arteries to the lungs] which led to gangrene and required amputation of first one then the other leg. During active treatment he received narcotics for which placebo injections were later substituted. Severe unremitting phantom limb pain was unrelieved by local measures and the neurosurgeon could only offer radical neurosurgery, which the patient declined. This man continued to take two daily injections of sterile saline solution, which satisfied him. He had become so dependent on them that he experienced great pain when they were omitted. Because of this man's underlying chronic disability it was decided to continue the placebos until such time as he might voluntarily relinquish them. (Leslie 1954)

It should be obvious even if you don't understand all the language that this was a very sick man who was in a lot of pain. One element of this case is particularly important and interesting. Phantom limb pain is a condition which seems very paradoxical, and yet leads to a much fuller understanding of what pain involves. It occasionally happens that people who have limbs amputated *can still feel them*; it is as if they are still there, and they can experience excruciating pain from such amputated limbs. Sometimes it feels as if the limb is grossly distorted; as if, for example, the leg were twisted up along the back pointing at the head.

What is most odd about this is the common-sense notion we all have that, for example, if I hit my thumb with a hammer, and it really hurts, the pain is in the thumb. It certainly feels that way. But the case of phantom limb pain indicates that such an obvious and sensible idea is wrong, or at least incomplete. Pain occurs primarily in the brain. Injury may occur to your thumb, but the pain is in the brain.

Pain, while unpleasant and even, sometimes, totally debilitating, is obviously a fundamental and extremely important process. If there was no particular information available to us as to the injuries we were sustaining, we might continue doing the things that are causing injury (indeed, sometimes we do that!). Pain is our way to tell ourselves to stop doing something dangerous or destructive. Pain can, however, sometimes become a very destructive messenger.

The primary concept of pain today is the "gate control theory" of Ronald Melzack and Patrick Wall (Melzack and Wall 1965). This theory says that certain small nerve fibers in the spinal cord conduct most pain signals, while larger nerve fibers conduct most other sensory information. When you hit your thumb with the hammer, the small fibers activate and open "neural gates" which allow messages to reach the brain; then you feel pain. Large fiber activity can close the gate, stopping the pain. So, if you put some ice cubes on your thumb, the sensory information ("cold") can trigger the large fibers to close the "pain gate" and stop the pain. These gates can also apparently be controlled from the other end of the system as well. So, if you are engaged in an exuberant touch-football game, you may get whacked on your leg hard enough to form a nasty bruise which you may not even notice until you get home and into the shower. On the other hand, you might get a paper cut turning the pages of a boring book which hurts enough that you quit reading. A generation ago Henry Beecher, who was to become one of the best-known researchers on the placebo effect, was an army surgeon in the Second World War; he noticed that soldiers with serious wounds often seemed not to be experiencing much pain. They would, however, complain when he gave them an antibiotic injection! (Beecher 1946) It is also clear that the gates which control pain (in part) can become confused – hence phantom limb pain.

In addition to these gate control mechanisms, there are other fascinating complications regarding the control or modulation of pain in the brain. Most striking are the endorphins, a class of neurotransmitters which act in the brain in essentially the same way as does morphine; the word "endorphin" is based on the notion of *endo*genous [internal] mo*rphine*. When the endorphins were discovered in the 1970s, there were passionate debates about the odd notion that the brain could produce substances to which it could become "addicted." Any orthopedist who treats athletes will tell you that many people with ruined feet, knees, hips, even sacroiliac joints, will just not stop running; they are addicted to their own endorphins, produced to control the pain of their exercise.

All of this is related to the experience of that poor man with two amputated legs. He apparently had become addicted to inert injections of saline solution. How ever could such a thing happen?

Placebo – and opiate – analgesia

There are two major forms of analgesics, or pain controllers. Some pain killers act "centrally" – that is, they affect pain over the whole body. The most global form of analgesic is the opiates like morphine, codeine, and related drugs which can reduce pain any place that it occurs in the body. As already noted, these drugs mimic the action of the endogenous opiates.

Another central form of analgesia is the "NSAIDs" – the non-steroidal anti-inflammatory drugs. These include aspirin, ibuprofen, naproxen, and another half-dozen related compounds. The way these drugs work is not fully clear, but it seems to involve the "prostaglandins." Prostaglandins are fats, or fatty acids, which are involved in the inflammatory response to injury and infection and are somehow engaged with the processes by which the body maintains its temperature. They are also instrumental in the production and maintenance of the mucous layer in the gut (which protects your stomach from digesting itself). Aspirin and the other NSAIDs inhibit the body's ability to produce prostaglandins, hence reducing the inflammatory response (and, apparently, pain), reducing fever, and reducing the efficiency of the protective layer in the gut (a common problem for people with arthritis – who take lots of NSAIDs – is often peptic ulcers). The physiological mechanisms and processes involved in the action of the NSAIDs are not very clear, but they are very important. (Three scientists – John Vane, Bengt Samuelsson and Sune Bergstrom – won the Nobel Prize in 1982 for discovering the prostaglandins.) These drugs are most effective for physical or muscular pains, bruises, and the like. They do not have much effect on, say, a stomach ache or intestinal pain. They also work, as we all know, for headaches.

In both these cases, the effect of the drug – NSAIDs or opiates – is quite general. That is, if you take ibuprofen for your football bruise, it will simultaneously ease the pain on your smashed thumb. By contrast, a drug like Novocaine has its effect only very locally, and if you were to treat your thumb with it, it wouldn't affect the bruise on your leg. Novocaine, or procaine hydrochloride, is a drug similar to cocaine in its structure which inhibits nerve impulses (it does so by inhibiting calcium in the nerve). There is a long list of similar drugs which also block such nerve action (perhaps the most exotic is curare) by inhibiting one or another part of nerve activity. While these two sets of mechanisms are analytically distinct, they are quite closely related.

Here is a brief account of how opiate analgesia works. There are a number of neurotransmitters involved, but among the most important are the endorphins. A way to think about them is this: neurotransmitters are rather like keys which fit into certain "locks" called receptor sites. When the endorphin fits into the receptor site and is activated (when "the key turns"), the pain stops. Because of a quite remarkable evolutionary history of their own, poppies can produce chemicals which mimic the action of these endorphins; the reasons for this are complex, but essentially the opiates act as poisons which protect the plants from being browsed by various animals and insects (the endorphins, and this whole process of pain control, are very widespread in nature). So, the first thing to notice is that it is not *only* endorphins which can activate these receptor sites; chemicals produced by plants can do it, too.

There is in this case another class of chemicals called antagonists which are very interesting. An opiate antagonist, like the drug naloxone, you can imagine to be like a blank key that you might get at a hardware store; if you get the right blank, but don't have it cut to match your key, you will be able to put it in the lock on the front door, but then you will run into problems. First, you won't be able to unlock the door with it, and second, you won't be able to use your regular key until you take the blank out of the door. Similarly, the antagonist will block the action of endorphins, but it will not have the effect of endorphins. Naloxone (trade name in the US is Narcan) is such an opiate antagonist; it is regularly used to treat people who have had drug overdoses. Simply put, if someone has taken any opiate, the effects can be reversed or diminished by giving a dose of naloxone.

In 1978, Jon Levine, Newton Gordon, and Howard Fields, all from the University of California in San Francisco, published an account of an extraordinary experiment. Working with young people who were having wisdom teeth removed, they gave their patients various drugs to treat the pain. Drugs were given double-blind through an intravenous drip so that no one knew who was getting what. Most patients were given placebo as their first pain treatment about two hours after the surgery. Then, an hour later, they were given another treatment, either a second placebo or naloxone. Although there were no differences in the pain reported by the two groups at the time of the second treatment, another hour later the patients who received naloxone reported significantly more pain than those who got a second placebo. Naloxone had reversed placebo analgesia.

The researchers reported the same data another way. They divided the patients into two groups, those who had a strong pain-relieving response to the initial placebo (the "placebo responders") and those who did not (the "placebo nonresponders"). They then looked at the response to naloxone in these two groups. The reduction in pain after receiving naloxone was significantly greater in the responders than in the nonresponders. Naloxone reversed the placebo effect in proportion to its size: big placebo effect, big reversal; small placebo effect, small reversal (Levine, Gordon, and Fields 1978).

There were problems with this study, which became extremely controversial. But it really marked a new day. No longer could anyone argue that "the placebo effect is all in your mind," you are just making something up, fooling yourself. Well, maybe you are making something up, but the something seems to be endorphins! There had been some research before this which pointed the way, but this was a turning point.

It was not a perfect experiment. For starters, there was no way to know if the placebo treatment really had any effect, since there was no group which received no treatment. There were lots of groups of patients, and only forty-seven subjects in the experiment, so the numbers were pretty small. The study was roundly criticized, but it did stimulate a significant amount of research by others. The results of various studies were conflicting. Some showed that while naloxone reversed some placebo analgesia, it didn't reverse all of it; some showed different results for "experimental pain" (pain induced in a laboratory) than for "clinical pain" (pain after surgery, for example) (Grevert, Albert, and Goldstein 1983); and there were indications that placebo effects and the effects of naloxone had different mechanisms (Gracely *et al.* 1983). The whole situation was quite confused, and while it seemed clear that something important was going on, research moved in different directions.

The Benedetti clarification

More recently, fortunately, that situation has changed. A team of researchers in Italy under the direction of Fabrizio Benedetti has done a series of experiments with placebo, naloxone and other neurotransmitters which have clarified much of the placebo-opiate connection. He carefully examined the earlier controversies, and designed a series of experiments which addressed all of the issues raised (Benedetti and Amanzio 1997). In one quite extraordinary experiment, he enrolled 340 healthy volunteers (Benedetti 1996). After being attached to a saline solution intravenous line in the right arm, they each were subjected to a standard form of experimentally induced pain – a tourniquet is placed on the left arm to limit blood flow, and the person has to squeeze a hand exerciser regularly for a short time. This causes a persistent pain which increases over time. Subjects were asked to rate the pain on a scale from 1 to 10, where 1 was "no pain at all" and 10 was "unbearable pain." When the individuals got to 7 on the scale, they were given a drug, administered through the intravenous drip. The advantage of this intravenous drip scheme was that subjects could be shown that they were receiving a drug, or one could be administered secretly, so that the subjects had no idea they were getting such treatments. Some results from the study are shown in Figure 8.1.

The outcome for a large group of sixty-seven subjects is shown in the figure in the line with the open squares. When these folks got to reporting 7 on the pain scale, they were given a secret injection of saline solution; the substance was inert, and they didn't know about it, so it had no meaning for them. This formed the "natural history" or "no treatment" group. In these people, the pain continued to increase over a period of about forty-five minutes, until they were saying the pain was roughly 10 on the scale, and the experiment was completed; the pain increased slowly but surely to the maximum bearable pain. In another group of ten (solid triangles on the graph), instead of getting a hidden dose of saline, they got a hidden dose of naloxone. This made no difference; their pain increased the same amount as those who got a hidden "placebo"; for this form of experimentally induced pain, naloxone does not affect pain.

Then the fun began. Benedetti wanted to see what the effect was of placebo responders to various secondary treatments. So 223 subjects were given a saline injection in full view when they got up to 7 on the pain scale, and they were told a very simple story: "I'm going to give you a painkiller. Your pain will subside after some minutes. Be calm and comfortable and

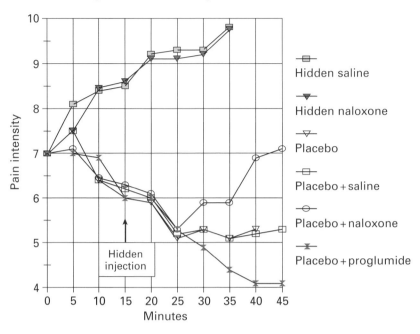

8.1   Elements of placebo analgesia (*Source*: Benedetti 1996)

report your pain sensation during the next minutes" (Benedetti 2000). Sixty of these people were clear placebo responders; rather than having their pain continue upward for the next hour, as it did in the control group, their pain decreased, and was rated as less than 7 fifteen minutes later. He divided the placebo responders into several subgroups and treated them in a variety of ways. One of these groups, shown by the open triangles on the graph, was given the visible injection of saline at time 0, and their pain started to decrease shortly thereafter. They were given no additional treatments, and their pain continued to lessen until it stabilized at about 5.1 on the scale, dramatically lower than the open square people who got no treatment that they were aware of; the only difference between the group marked "no treatment" and the group marked "placebo" is that the second group knew they got a drug and the first didn't know it, although they got the same drug (an inert one). Placebo treatment can dramatically reduce pain compared to no treatment, but only if the subjects know it is happening. It is not the placebo itself that reduces the pain, which makes perfect sense since it is inert. It is the *knowledge* of the placebo that does the trick.

Benedetti then studied three more groups which showed a placebo response to the first injection (at "time zero"). Each of these groups received a second *hidden* injection fifteen minutes after the first open injection. One group (open squares, labeled "placebo + saline" on the figure) received a secret injection of saline solution after fifteen minutes. You can see on the graph that this group has essentially the same reaction as the placebo group; the pain decreases and then stabilizes at about 5.1. A hidden dose of inert drug which the subject doesn't know about doesn't do anything.

In another group (open circles on the graph, labeled "placebo + naloxone"), we see the same result which Dr. Levine and his colleagues showed in their experiment: the pain reported starts to increase as the opiate antagonist ("blank key") naloxone reverses the placebo effect. The pain of these subjects never gets all the way up to 10 on the scale, but it might continue to increase if they continued the experiment for another hour or so, or it may be that naloxone only reverses some portion (half?) of the meaning response.

The last line on the graph requires a bit more elaboration. The opioid pain response is very complex, far more complex than I have indicated here. There is another neurotransmitter called "cholecystokinin" (CCK). CCK acts to *inhibit* the action of the endorphins. Pain control in the central nervous system is a complex balancing act, with some things (like the endorphins) reducing pain, and some things (like CCK) enhancing it. CCK not only inhibits the action of the endorphins, but it also inhibits the action of morphine.

But just as naloxone blocks the action of the endorphins, there is a chemical called proglumide which blocks the action of CCK! Proglumide, then, *enhances* the effect of morphine by getting in the way of an endogenous chemical (CCK) that increases pain. And this is what accounts for the last line on our graph. This group of subjects (solid Xs on the graph, labeled "placebo + proglumide") showed a significant response to the open placebo treatment at time zero, and their pain started to decrease. After fifteen minutes, they received a hidden injection of proglumide. Rather than leveling off at 5.1 as did the other placebo-treated groups, their pain continued down to nearly 4 on the scale.

These elegant experiments clearly demonstrate that inert placebo treatments presented to people in pain as a "painkiller" can substantially reduce pain compared either 1) to a group receiving no such placebo (a "natural history group"), or 2) to a group receiving the inert treatment hidden so they don't know it. This meaning response (to the words "here's a painkiller") can be reversed with naloxone, and enhanced with proglumide.

Placebo analgesia without placebos

In a more recent study, Dr. Benedetti and his colleagues gave surgical patients one of several pain treatments appropriate for their surgery – narcotics or aspirin-like medicines. Some patients got their pain medication secretly, through an intravenous line. Other patients got the same kind of medication openly, from an injection by a doctor or nurse; they were told "it was a powerful painkiller increasing [their] pain tolerance." Patients were asked how much pain they were experiencing, and were given medication (openly or otherwise) until the pain reported was half what it was at the beginning. Patients who knew they were getting the medication required substantially less medication than those who didn't know it (Amanzio *et al.* 2001). The fact of experiencing the medication made it work better. In a variation on this experiment, the researchers (ethically unable to do this with surgical patients) induced pain in volunteers in a laboratory; they gave them analgesics either surreptitiously or openly, and found the same results as in the clinical situation: subjects who were given open injections by a clinician needed less medication to get pain relief than did the secretly medicated patients. They were then able to block this increased pain relief with naloxone.

This looks like the placebo effect, but it's important to recognize there were no placebos involved. Everyone in these studies received active medication; the difference was their experience of getting the treatment. In commenting on the study, pain researcher Donald Price said that although the increase in pain relief in this study experienced by the openly treated patients was, by itself, probably not clinically significant, "both pain research scientists and the pharmaceutical industry go to the ends of the earth to make improvements [to existing drugs] of this magnitude. Adding one or two sentences to each pain treatment might help to produce them" (Price 2001). He is clearly right, and what we have here is "two little sentences," or a "meaning response," with no placebos in sight.

Of pain, poetry, music, and love

What do we learn from these remarkable experiments? At one level, it seems clear not only that the imposition of meaning on an inert treatment for pain can reduce the pain, but also that we can see there are "real," "biological," mechanisms which might, to some degree or other, "account" for the pain reduction. Moreover, this biological process can be both blocked, at least partially, with naloxone, and it can be enhanced with proglumide. Of course, there is no hint in this remarkable work about how this might happen, any more than we know what exactly happens between the instant when I *decide* to tell you that I love you, and when I actually form the consonants and vowels which come (haltingly?) out of my mouth and I actually *say* "I love you." But in this case of placebo analgesia, we seem to know for certain that "something" is really happening "in there" (and for which, in the latter case of my profession of love, we'd best wait a few months and see). Placebo analgesia seems simultaneously to be a biological and meaningful process, perhaps not unlike love.

There are dissenters, and some not to take lightly. Patrick Wall has already been mentioned here as the co-creator of the gate control theory of pain. In a paper published in 1993 (after the work of Levine, Grevert, and Gracely, but before the work of Benedetti) he wrote this paragraph which I quote at length. He referred to Levine's work, and noted that it

gave the placebo instant respectability in twentieth century terms, and liberated it from [many] doubts and denials.... [But] the logic of this reasoning for the admission of the placebo to polite society is zero. If a newspaper headline read: 'Scientists discover the origin of music and poetry' followed by an article showing that music could not be performed when curare prevented the effect of acetyl choline released from the motor axons [and the performer was, thereby, paralyzed], one would not be overwhelmed by the insight into the nature of music and poetry. Similarly, it is not clear what insight into the overall placebo phenomenon is provided by showing that some link in the machinery involves endorphins. (Wall 1993:97)

But I disagree with Dr. Wall, even though I see his point. Given the long history of resistance and opposition to the reality of meaning responses in the Western world (though not by Dr. Wall!), it is extremely helpful to see that there really is something like machinery there![29] That real biological processes – which can be inhibited or enhanced by particular biological agents – are involved at all may help others to see that *meaning* is not simply some wooly fantasy from the fringe, some airy pipedream, or otherworldly spiritism. Human biology is comprised of neurons, neurotransmitters and synapses; but it is also comprised of meaning, experience, knowledge and practice.

The cultural biology of pain; WASPS, Jews and Italians

It seems to be the case, too, that this experience, knowledge, and information can occur in patterned ways in the world so that people with different cultures experience pain differently; the different meanings in their lives mean that their pain processes work differently. There is long-standing

[29] Dr. Wall died in August, 2001, at the age of 76, just as I was finishing this chapter. He was a great scientist who will be deeply missed.

evidence that people from different ethnic groups (different cultures) experience pain – both acute and chronic pain – differently.

In 1952, anthropologist Mark Zborowski published a landmark paper titled "Cultural Components in Responses to Pain"; years later, he published a book expanding on his earlier paper titled *People in Pain* (Zborowski 1952, 1969). These works were based on years of research at a Veterans Administration Hospital in the Bronx, New York. Working with men, all military veterans, he probed peoples' responses to pain, their attitudes toward doctors, medication, and hospitalization, and so on. He studied these reactions among people of different backgrounds and cultures; in his first paper, he focused on what he called "Old Americans" – essentially White Anglo-Saxon Protestants (WASPS), people whose families had been living in the United States for three or more generations – as well as several groups of more recent immigrants, particularly Jews and Italians. In the later book, he added a consideration of Irish immigrants. About two-thirds were working-class men who did physical labor, while the remainder were primarily engaged in small business or professional work as teachers or the like; most were suffering from serious, long-term back pain, most with herniated disks and spinal lesions of one sort or another. He found that Jews and Italians had quite different attitudes to pain than did Old Americans. Doctors and nurses told him that Jews and Italians were alike in being excessively emotional in their responses to pain compared to the Old Americans, who were much more stoical. He found that while indeed the Jews and Italians tended to be very vocal about their pain, the Italians were much more eager than the Jews to have the pain treated, and, once it was controlled, they seemed quite satisfied with the situation; whereas even when the pain was controlled, Jews continued to worry about it, seeing pain as a harbinger of more dangers to come. He argued that while the Italians were "present oriented" with respect to pain, the Jews were more "future oriented." The Old Americans were also more future-oriented, but much more optimistic than the Jews. The Old Americans, seeing the body in a rather mechanical way, seemed to imagine that, under the care of competent professionals, the pain would diminish; the Jews imagined that treating the pain was only hiding a serious harbinger of real danger. When pain was severe, he found, Jews and Italians preferred to be surrounded by people – families, friends, doctors – while the Old Americans withdrew from society and wanted to be alone. In his book, Zborowski added a consideration of Irish immigrants, whom he described as being similar to the Old Americans in many ways but worrying much more about the long-term significance of their illnesses, and in this way being more like the Jews. Other factors also were at play; he noted, for example, that working men were more concerned with back pain, while the more "intellectual" men tended to be more concerned about headaches. He made two very interesting conclusions:

1) Similar reactions to pain manifested by members of different ethno-cultural groups do not necessarily reflect similar attitudes to pain. 2) Reactive patterns similar in terms of their manifestations may have different functions and serve different purposes in different cultures (Zborowski 1952:24).

In the terms we have used throughout this book, Zborowski is saying that essentially the same pain has quite different meanings in different cultures, and this shapes the individual's experience of it.

What is the source of the experience, knowledge and information that mediate these pain responses? Obviously, everyone grows up following his own trajectory, with this event preceding that one, this sad experience following that happy one. For an anthropologist, it is apparent that this is not simply an individual's experience, however. In different places and times, people grow up in different cultures, with dramatically different expectations about life, with extremely different customs and values, knowing very different things about the world. Culture is a complex topic, and a highly contested one which generates enormous controversy among scholars. One of the most striking things about culture is how invisible it is to us most of the time, at least until we come in contact with a different one. So, for example, in Chapter 6, I briefly described the "A + 2b" formula for American meals. We never think of ourselves following such rules (or breaking them) until we see people following different rules. One of the reasons that the concept of culture is so contested and controversial, I think, is because these matters of culture are experienced by all of us as moral matters of right vs. wrong, of good vs. bad. So, we might say, "Hmmm. That was a *good* meal" or "What's the *right* sauce to put on this fish?" And when we find people eating things we don't eat (puppies, horses, grubs), we usually first have a strong emotional reaction ("Sheesh, that's disgusting!") followed by a moral one ("It's just wrong to eat horses"). The concept of culture makes it more difficult to come so quickly to such moral judgments. It soon becomes clear that the guy in the other culture has the same sort of ideas about you. It is not comfortable being labeled immoral because you just ate a baloney sandwich. But it also allows us to imagine the reaction of the person whose diet upset us so much a few minutes ago ("puppies, horses").

The biggest analytical problem here is that, while on the one hand, such cultural matters are the most important things in our lives, there are also enormous areas of overlap and commonality among human lives, wherever you go. Customs like marriage, inheritance, religion and so on are universal; of course the details may vary, and they may vary dramatically. But these things will always be present, even if they are in any one place or time highly contentious. In contemporary American culture, apparently simple matters of diet are extremely contested. There are vegetarians of several types who often disagree deeply with one another about what are the proper things to eat. There are "ovo-lacto vegetarians" and "vegans," for example; I know a number of vegetarians who eat chicken; at the moment, my vegetarian daughter eats fish. There are highly secular American Jews who are scientists, or journalists, or doctors who might consider the story of Adam and Eve to be a lovely myth (and nothing more than that), who simply cannot force themselves to eat a pork chop. So maybe there *isn't* an American food culture; there are just 250 million different people, and they are all wrong about diet but me.

Of course there is an American food culture, and a religious culture, and a property culture, and all the rest. Australian aborigine cuisine will look as odd to a red-meat-eating American as it will to a vegan American.

Electric shock and other tortures

As we have seen, there is interesting evidence to show that these cultural factors can influence things as intimate and (apparently) biological as pain. Other studies have had results similar to Zborowski's. In a series of experiments in the 1960s, Bernard Tursky and Richard Sternbach showed a number of interesting differences in the way people from different ethnic groups (Yankee [= "Old American" = WASP], Irish, Jewish, and Italian) responded to electric shock (Sternbach and Tursky 1965; Tursky and Sternbach 1967). They started from a position similar to Zborowski's: "Yankees have a phlegmatic, matter of fact orientation toward pain; Jews express a concern for the implications of pain and distrust palliatives; Italians express a desire for pain relief and the Irish inhibit expression of suffering and concern for the implications of pain" (Tursky and Sternbach 1967). The researchers associated these differences with a series of other differences in various measures of the activity of the autonomic nervous system, like heart rate, galvanic skin potential and resistance, and body temperature. For example, the Irish subjects showed a substantial (and statistically significant) difference in their galvanic skin resistance which was much lower than the other groups. This, they say, "is associated with their considerable anxiety which they feel constrained not to verbalize or express overtly." Psychologists generally interpret increased conductance of (or reduced resistance to) electricity through the skin as a measure of anxiety and inhibition or conflict – in this case, both. These experiments showed that there were additional biological variations between different cultural groups in response to the same stimulus – pain – which had different meanings for the different groups. These authors also noted significant variability within each of these groups in these physiological measures, but there were group differences as well.

By the late 1960s, there were enough studies of this sort that a review was possible (Wolff and Langley 1968). These authors, respectively a clinical psychologist and an anthropologist, concluded that, first, it was "quite clear from [several] studies . . . that cultural factors in terms of attitudinal variables, whether explicit or implicit, do indeed exert significant influences on pain perception." They were much less optimistic on a series of studies that were interested not in the reaction to pain, but to the actual sensation of pain, which we will consider briefly further on in this chapter.

Probably the best study of culture and pain was done in the mid-1980s by Maryann Bates and several colleagues (Bates, Edwards, and Anderson 1993). Bates studied 372 patients from six ethnic groups at a chronic pain clinic in Massachusetts. Most of these people, like those in Zborowski's study, had long-term debilitating back pain, although others had arthritis, or other sorts of neurological conditions. She gave a comprehensive test to determine the intensity of the pain that the patients experienced, and then attempted to see what other factors might have varied along with the pain intensity. Most of the things which differentiated the patients – gender, education, age, medical diagnosis, medication history, and so on – had no relationship to the intensity of pain the people reported. Three factors – age cohort, ethnic group affiliation, and locus of control (LOC) – did vary with reported pain. The oldest patients, over the age of 60, reported the lowest levels of pain (note that this is all relative: these were all people suffering a lot of pain); the youngest patients were in the middle; and the middle-aged patients, between 41 and 60, reported the most. While these differences were statistically significant, they weren't very large.

Figure 8.2 shows the total pain scores for the six ethnic groups. The obvious difference is between the Hispanics and all the rest; but controlling for other variables (age, locus of control), two different sets emerge (Hispanics, Italians and Irish on the one hand; Old Americans, French Canadians and Polish on the other), with the members of each set being alike one another and different from the other set.

The most interesting aspect of this study is the role of "locus of control." Locus of control is a term to describe the way in which people see forces in the world working. There are two possible locuses of control: internal and external. People with an internal locus of control see themselves as in control of the world they live in; they can change the world and have

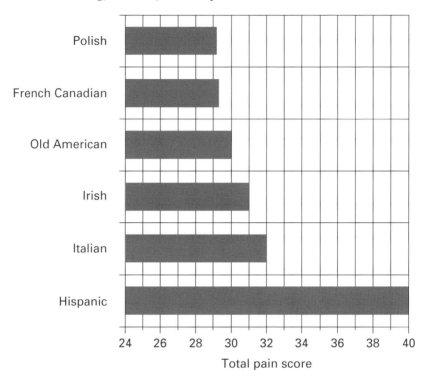

8.2   Cultural variation in chronic pain perception (*Source*: Bates *et al.*
1993)

power over it. People with an external locus of control see the world as
controlling them; they are subject to the forces of other people, chance, or
of "fate." Obviously, both conditions exist at the same time; I determine if
I will brush my teeth this morning or not, but I also recognize that there is
precious little I can do about the Chinese government's one-child policy,
or the weather. But the proportion of things which individuals put in each
category can vary quite dramatically, and this factor has been shown to
be related to a number of different aspects of health and stress.

In Bates' study, people with internal locus of control (regardless of
ethnic group or anything else) had lower pain intensity scores than those
with high scores (30.4 vs 36.9). This pattern was true in four of the six
ethnic groups, but in two of them (Old American, Polish) it was reversed:
the internal locus of control people expressed more pain than the external
types. Although Bates couldn't analyze it precisely, she reports that many
people in the study reported that the experience of severe chronic pain
changed their sense of control of their lives; where before they had more

sense of control than they did now, the experience of pain about which nothing could be done had changed that. Since the researchers met the people at the chronic pain clinic, they had no way to measure the locus of control before the pain had begun, so they couldn't test whether this changed in systematic ways as a result of different ethnic groups. Bates writes

Uniformly... [Hispanics] had significantly higher levels of interference with work and daily activities [due to pain], believed most strongly that as long as they had pain their lives would remain unhappy, reported that they express their pain more frequently and emotionally, and reported significantly higher degrees of worries, anger and tension associated with their pain. The [Italians were] consistently second highest in all of these response categories. [The Polish] were almost always lowest in each.

From Figure 8.2 you will recall that the Hispanics come first in reported pain intensity, the Italians second, and the Polish last.

Conclusions

Consider, finally, this eloquent statement about pain from a dentist (McGrath 1994):

Pain is a complex, multidimensional perception that varies in quality, strength, duration, location, and unpleasantness. The strength and unpleasantness of pain is neither simply nor directly related to the nature and extent of tissue damage. Even newborn infants may experience different pains from the same stimulus, because of the differences in the situations in which it is administered. Pain experiences can range from an inability to perceive pain, regardless of the strength of stimulation, to the actual perception of pain in a limb that has been amputated. The perception of, expression of, and reaction to pain are influenced by genetic, developmental, familial, psychological, social and cultural variables. Psychological factors, such as the situational and emotional factors that exist when we experience pain, can profoundly alter the strength of these perceptions. Attention, understanding, control, expectations, and [its] aversive significance can affect pain perceptions. Consequently, the understanding of pain requires not only understanding of the nociceptive system, but recognition and control of the many environmental and psychological factors that modify human pain perceptions.

This is, clearly, a very complicated situation where we are seeing the world dimly, but it seems pretty clear that what people think and know about pain – what pain means – varies systematically among people of different backgrounds, ages, and attitudes, and that difference in meaning affects the ways they perceive their bodies, their illnesses, and probably their cures. But, no one said it was going to be easy.

9 "More research is needed": The cases of "adherence" and "self-reported health"

I have tried throughout this book to make a coherent case, accounting for as much material as I could. One great value of the concept of the meaning response is that it allows us to look carefully and creatively at things which, to now, have seemed mysterious and puzzling, to make sense of them, and to see how they relate to one another. Another value is that it lets us connect together under one umbrella things which previously seemed to be unrelated, or simply off the charts. Among those are the research on "adherence" and on "self-rated health." I am confident that these are important instances of the effects of meaning on human health; but the details of how this is the case are not at all clear.

Adherence and survival

One of the strangest instances of the meaning response involves the notion of "adherence," also called "compliance." In the late 1960s, a major study was carried out involving several drugs including one called clofibrate which lowers the levels of cholesterol and triglycerides in the blood. The study was an attempt to learn if this treatment actually reduced the rate of mortality from heart attacks. The patients in the study were all men between the ages of 30 and 64 who showed evidence of having had a myocardial infarction (a heart attack) in the previous three months. It was a very large study with thousands of patients; 1,103 men were assigned to the clofibrate group and 2,789 were assigned to the placebo group. The men were followed for a minimum of five years; the study ended in 1974. The study showed that there was no difference in survival five years after the patient's heart attack for the two groups: 20.0% of the men taking clofibrate had died, and 20.9% of the men taking the placebo had died. This is not a statistically significant difference, and could be expected to occur by chance half the time (p = .55). One of the things that the researchers had watched very carefully was how much of their medicine the men had taken. They had to take a lot of medicine – for most of the five-year period, they had to take three capsules three times a day. Two-thirds of the men took more than 80% of their pills – these were said to be good "adherers" – they adhered well to the therapeutic regimen.

The researchers noticed that men who took most of their prescribed clofibrate, more than 80% of what was prescribed, did better than the men who took less. After five years, only 15.7% of the good adherers had died, while 22.5% of the poor adherers had died. The message seems to be "take all your medicine." But it is more complicated than this because the same thing happened with the placebo patients. Men who took more than 80% of their placebos had a five-year mortality rate of 16.4% while those who took less had a mortality rate of 25.8% (CDPRG 1980). The second message seems to be "take all your placebos."

This result has been seen in other studies as well. People with cancer often experience serious infections after they have had chemotherapy. In the early 1980s, researchers enrolled 150 cancer patients (mostly young people; the median age was 17) in a study of antibiotics given after each cycle of chemotherapy. About half the patients got antibiotics and half got matching placebos; 22% of antibiotic patients, and 27% of placebo patients, got infections or fevers. About 61% of drug patients were judged to have had excellent compliance with their therapy as were somewhat more placebo patients who had higher levels of compliance. "Patients with excellent compliance had a lower incidence of fever or infections than those with good or poor compliance, regardless of whether they received drug... or placebo... "(Pizzo et al. 1983:129). These differences were large and highly statistically significant (in either case, they might occur by chance one time in 1,000). But they were also clinically significant. Among patients taking antibiotics, only 18% of good adherers had infections or fever while among poor adherers, 53% had them (three times as many). Among the placebo patients, 32% of good adherers had infections, but 64% of poor adherers did (twice as many). So it's clear that "antibiotics work," and protect against infections. But so does taking all your drug, or placebo, as the case may be.

Similar findings come from a study of chlorpromazine (Thorazine) for people suffering the demons of schizophrenia (Hogarty and Goldberg 1973). This complex study was looking at the interaction of drug treatment and certain forms of psychotherapy. People with this awful disease were stabilized in the hospital with drug treatment. They were subsequently released to outpatient clinics which followed them in their normal lives. Of the drug treated patients, 32% relapsed into schizophrenia as did 73% of the placebo-treated patients. In the previous example we saw that antibiotics effectively prevent infection in chemotherapy patients, and in this study, Thorazine is shown to be an effective drug for treating schizophrenia. But, of drug patients who took their medications regularly, only about 13% relapsed compared to 57% of those who took their medications irregularly. Of the placebo patients who took their "medications" regularly, about 40% relapsed compared with 80% for those who took fewer of their pills. Only half as many "placebo adherent" patients relapsed as did "placebo less adherent" patients. Again, we see that it's important to "take all your placebos."

Another study has also shown taking all your placebos can protect against heart attack. In a study of the data derived from an important project examining the effect of the beta-blocker propranalol on heart attack, over 2,000 men were randomly assigned to receive the drug or placebo. These men had already had a serious heart attack before being enrolled in the study. After a year, 1.4% of men who had taken more than three-quarters of their beta blockers had died from second heart attacks while 4.2% of those who had taken less medicine had died; three times as many with poor compliance died. And, after a year, 3% of men taking all their placebos died while 7% of those with poorer compliance had died; 2.3 times as many with poor compliance died. These researchers had quite detailed information on these men – the medical and social histories, their smoking and drinking behavior, etc. – which they factored into the equation. Adjusting for all these factors made an appreciable difference; the adjustments lowered the odds favoring compliant patients from 3 to 2.8 (Horwitz *et al.* 1990).

A few years later, some of these same researchers showed that the same thing held for the 602 women who had been enrolled in the beta blocker trial. Four and a half percent of women who took all their propranolol had died after a year compared with 8.7% of those who took less medication; among placebo patients, 6.8% of good adherers, but 19% of poor adherers, died. Again, adjusting for all the various risk factors made no difference (Gallagher, Viscoli, and Horwitz 1993). In these two studies, the proportion of poor adherers to medicine was the same for men (7.3%) and women (8.7%). In a more recent study from Canada, poor adherers to drug and placebo were twice as likely to have died of various cardiac failures than were adherent patients two years after the study began (Irvine *et al.* 1999).

These studies are very confusing to scientists. They simply don't know what to make of them. There is a problem with the data from an analytic point of view. The patients have not been randomized to the conditions of being adherent or not. So, scientists reason, they must be two different kinds of people from the start. For example, "*Obviously*, there must be characteristics differentiating between good and poor adherers (e.g., alcohol use and abuse, behavioral characteristics, or socioeconomic status) not accounted for in the variables assessed in [this study]" (CDPRG 1980:1040; my italics). The problem is that, in the other studies, where these things *were* taken into account, they don't explain the difference. Good adherers to drugs or placebos do better than poor adherers regardless of behavior or economic status. And no one knows why.

Health perception and survival

The situation is very similar regarding the effects of what is called "health perception." In several dozen studies it has been shown that, especially (but not only) for older people, one of the very best predictors of future longevity or mortality is the answer that people give to *one* question: "In general, would you say your health is: excellent, very good, good, fair, [or] poor." One of the earlier studies showed that, among a sample of over 3,000 older Canadians in Manitoba, those who rated their health as "excellent" in 1971 were 2.9 times as likely to still be alive in 1977 than were those who rated their health as "poor." This bit of information – self-rated health – was a better indicator of mortality than any other thing except for age itself (people over 90 have a low life expectancy regardless of their sense of their own health). This "subjective" measure was better than a long series of other "objective" measures based on a detailed examination and history taken by a physician. The individuals' own ("subjective") assessments were much better predictors of mortality than were the doctors' ("objective") assessments (Mossey and Shapiro 1982).

Similarly, nearly 7,000 Californians who were over 60 were asked the same question in 1965. Nine years later, adjusting for their ages, men who had rated their health as excellent were 2.33 times as likely to be alive as were men who rated their health as poor; women were 5.1 times as likely to be alive when they rated their health as excellent (Kaplan and Camacho 1983). In a follow-up study seventeen years after the study began, the combined, age-adjusted advantage for those who had rated their health as excellent remained: those who professed excellent health were 2.3 times as likely to be alive as were those who rated it to be poor (Kaplan *et al.* 1987).

The most subtle work on this issue has been done by Ellen Idler of Rutgers University and her colleagues. She has tried to tease out just what it is that causes this effect, trying to find what personal characteristics people have who report excellent health compared to those who don't. She had similar results in a study of 2,800 men and women over 65 living in New Haven, Connecticut (Idler and Kasl 1991). Men who rated their health as excellent were nearly 7 times less likely to die within four years than those who rated it as poor; women with excellent self-rated health were 3.1 times less likely to die as those with poor self-rated health. Idler included a whole range of other factors in her analysis; among them were the subjects' disease history, age, smoking behavior, and weight; their medical history: whether they had recently been hospitalized or in a nursing home, and the number and kind of medications they took; the support they had available, the number of friends and family, their religious activity and religiosity, their attitudes and moods. Several of these (age, smoking) predicted some portion of four-year mortality, but none had as much effect as did global self assessment of health. "Self-rated health," Idler writes, "appears to have a unique, predictive, and thus far inexplicable relationship with mortality."

How can we understand adherence and global health rating?

Idler considers two possible explanations for self-rated health; I will describe them in reverse order. Second, she says in effect, people describing their own health may just be extremely knowledgeable about it. The question of how you rate your health "may be eliciting an estimate of subjective life expectancy, based on calculations that could take in a broad range of data known only to the respondent: his or her family's chronic disease history, how long-lived or short-lived were the parents and grandparents, a close identification with a relative with whom the respondent shared a physical resemblance, health condition, or life style." In the terms we have used, Idler is describing something people "know." One of the most common ways that researchers assess "health perception" is through a questionnaire known as "SF-36" – a form with thirty-six questions on it. In one version, the first of the thirty-six questions is the one about global health, and the responses are strung across the page. Below each response ("Excellent," "Very good," etc.) there is a little circle you have to fill in with a pencil (Medical Outcomes Trust and Ware 2000). This is, perhaps, the shortest story you will ever write: one little circle. This experience – filling in the dot – is even shorter and punchier than that experienced by the students writing about their traumas in the studies by Pennebaker. In both cases, one has to make a judgment based on a lifetime of personal experience of what's important, and then to tell a story. One wonders how many million times someone has walked into his psychiatrist's office, sat down, and been asked "So, how are you this week?" And you tell your story. The story on SF-36 is shorter than that, but, even in its remarkable simplicity ("In general, would you say your health is: _____"), it is much more global and compelling, sort of

Shakespearean or Dostoyevskian. And it is, of course, especially for older people, exquisitely meaningful.

Recall that Idler had two possible explanations: "The first [possibility] is that the perception of health status has some beneficial or detrimental effect on the individual's subsequent experience of morbidity [sickness, or illness]. In this case people who report good health despite medical findings or, conversely, people whose health complaints are apparently unjustified, may actually alter their risk of mortality by bringing their health status into line with their self-perceptions." That is, filling in that little circle on the form may be some sort of self-fulfilling prophecy. It may change the future in the same way the widely advertised brand name on the tablet does for the woman with a headache (even though, perhaps, the tablet is inert); or it may change the future pain experienced by people given an injection of sterile saline solution by someone who thinks that just *maybe* they are getting fentanyl.

Idler says these two possibilities – the knowledge option and the self-fulfilling prophecy option – are "logically alternative." But of course they needn't be mutually exclusive. We have seen that it is quite possible for very modest sorts of engagement with meaning to have significant impact on human health and healing. Telling the world's very shortest story – "my health is . . . *excellent*" (fill in the circle) – may be another case.

The adherence case is even more opaque. But "taking a pill" is not dissimilar from filling in the dot on the questionnaire; each time you take a pill, you experience a little bit of the whole medical experience you had when you first received it. The dark cloud can represent the whole onrushing storm, because it's part of the storm; "counting noses," or "military brass," like the dark cloud, are cases where a part of something (the nose; the insignia on the hat; the cloud) *represents*, or *stands for*, or *means* something else (you; ranking officers; the storm). These are technically examples of *synecdoche*, representations which literally are meaningless or nonsensical, but figuratively can be very compelling. In some senses, a pill, too, is a synecdoche, in that it can recall the whole medical encounter. We have already seen that four placebos can work better than two; so it doesn't seem a great jump to see that 100% of the placebos (or drugs, for that matter) might work better than three-quarters of them. But of course, that doesn't tell us why some people die and some don't. It is doubtless the case that "more research is needed."

10 Other approaches: learning, expecting, and conditioning

I have tried to make a coherent presentation of an argument for meaning in medicine. It should come as no surprise to know that, gently phrased, "others disagree." This is a highly contentious and rancorous business sometimes. In this chapter, I want to show some areas in healing which are similar to the meaning response, but can't be explained by it. I also want to compare the meaning response with other approaches which might overlap with what I have described, and to suggest that the differences may be as much semantic as anything else. In any case, here are some limitations and challenges to the meaning response.

"Conditioning" placebo effects

Dr. Fabrizio Benedetti has done another quite remarkable experiment (Benedetti *et al.* 1999). It's not easy to explain, so watch carefully. One of the dangers of narcotic painkillers is that one of their "side effects" is to depress respiration; they reduce your ability to breathe. In this experiment, sixty people with lung cancer were having surgery to remove portions of the lung. After the surgery, they were given a narcotic (buprenorphine) through a saline drip. For three days, they would receive a fairly large dose of the narcotic in the morning, and then a much lower dose throughout the day. Dr. Benedetti measured the patient's respiration each day just before the morning dose of narcotic, and then an hour later; he measured the volume of air (in liters) that the patient breathed in a minute. Each day, the patients breathed about 9 liters of air per minute before the injection and about 7.5 or 8 liters per minute an hour later. On the fourth day, patients are usually pain free and, ordinarily, don't receive any more medication for pain. But in this case, they received one more treatment. The patients were divided into five groups of twelve. The patients in three of the groups were told that they were going to receive one more dose of narcotic. In one of these groups, the patients were actually given a dose of placebo after being told they would get the narcotic. Their breathing was tested before the placebo, and an hour after. The amount of air that they breathed dropped from 9 liters per minute to 8. The injection produced a "placebo side effect"! Two of the groups were told they would get the narcotic again, but were instead given (a small or large dose of) naloxone, the opiate antagonist we have heard of before. In the group with the large dose, the amount of air they breathed was the same an hour after the injection as it was before. The "side effect" could be blocked by naloxone (the smaller dose had a smaller effect). Hang on now, we are almost done. In the fourth group, the patients were given the same breathing test as all the others, but no placebos, no naloxone, no treatment at all. Their breathing was the same both times. The same was true with the last group which got a hidden naloxone injection; their breathing was normal both times. The day *before* surgery, all of the patients had been given a placebo treatment, and were told that it was the same narcotic they would get after surgery; their breathing was checked both before and an hour after the placebo injection. The breathing was normal both times, and it did not drop.

A few more details are useful here. Although the respiratory depression here was clearly measurable, it was not so significant that the patients felt short of breath; they did not know that their breathing was depressed. And on top of that, they didn't generally know that these narcotics *caused* respiratory depression. They knew that narcotics were painkillers, but not that they were respiratory depressants.

What can we learn from this experiment? An amusing but somewhat simplistic interpretation might be that placebos can have "side effects."[30] We have already discussed the ambiguity of the notion of a drug's "side effect"; my sense is that drugs have effects on physiology, some of them desirable, and some not desirable. What is desirable and undesirable can change with circumstance: diphenhydramine ("Benadryl") makes you sleepy while it dries up your sinuses: if you want an antihistamine, this one makes you sleepy; if you want a sleeping tablet, this one gives you a dry mouth. In the case of opiates, it is clear that vertebrates have evolved a complex pain control mechanism involving endogenous opiates which both reduce pain and depress respiration. I don't know why the two are linked, but they seem to be. Perhaps, in an evolutionary context, reduced respiration means that you simply can't be as active as you might be otherwise, and rest is good for you while you are in pain. This experiment, then, indicates that the biological processes which can be triggered by meaningful experiences can be complex and robust.

But there is more to it than that. Notice that, so far as can be told from the description of the experiment, the patients didn't know that

---

[30] Nina Etkins has written a masterful paper about "side effects" in a cross-cultural context (Etkin 1992).

respiration decreased when they were given the drug; they didn't expect or know that respiration would be depressed. The treatments clearly had meaning ("narcotics are powerful painkillers"), but they did not have the meaning "narcotics repress respiration," even though that's true. Yet the people who were given an inert medication on the final day and were told it was a painkiller had a significant drop in respiration anyway (they did not have a significant drop in pain because, by then, they were not in pain any more). This drop in respiration did not happen on the day before surgery, before the patients had "learned" it. Dr. Benedetti interprets this as evidence that we are seeing the effect of "conditioning." What does this mean?

The best evidence of conditioning comes from studies on animals. The classic experiment involved "Pavlov's dogs." Dr. Pavlov was a famous Russian physiologist who, around the turn of the century, did a series of classic experiments on learning. He noticed that sometimes dogs would begin salivating even before the food was put in the bowls. So he started ringing a bell when he fed the dogs. After a while, the dogs would salivate when the bell rang. One can presume that the dogs didn't "know" that the bell "meant" food, that is, that the reactions were not cognitive ones involving understanding or meaning.

If that's what is happening in the case of Dr. Benedetti's experiment, then this is *not* a case of the meaning response, since the patients didn't know that one of the consequences of their treatment was respiratory repression. The patients were "conditioned" to reduce their respiration. They seem to have learned it in more or less the same way that Pavlov's dogs learned to salivate when they heard the bell ringing.

In my view, this is a very unusual experiment. Others disagree, and say that such conditioning accounts for most, or maybe even all, of the placebo effect (Wickramasekera 1980; Ader 1997). It is clear that, in a laboratory, one can condition animals to do quite remarkable things. Robert Ader has done what is probably the most interesting work on this issue. He found that when rats were given a drug which suppressed their immune response along with a particular sweet flavoring, he could subsequently suppress their immune systems with the sweet flavoring alone (Ader and Cohen 1975). He has subsequently suggested that, for someone who has to take regular doses of powerful or expensive drugs, one could randomly replace some portion of them with inert tablets, and the same effect would be achieved as if she took all of them. But this has not been tested in people. Of course, people in such a situation would know that they were taking drugs, and would be as subject to the meaning response as anyone else, so there is no reason to believe that this would be due to conditioning. Dr. Wall (of the "gate control" theory of pain discussed earlier) argues that there is no convincing evidence for conditioning in adult humans, and that "it may be that the passionately maintained differences between cognitive and conditioned responses will collapse" (Wall 1993). I think there may be a little bit of evidence for such conditioning (Dr. Benedetti's study with which we started this chapter) which shows that it is possible. But people come into any study or healing encounter with a lifetime of experience and knowledge of illness and healing – with a whole reservoir of meaning – which cannot easily be evaded.

Dr. Ader has written "there is, I believe, considerable heuristic value in viewing a pharmacotherapeutic regimen as a series of conditioning trials" (Ader 1997:159). Each time you take a pill, Dr. Ader might say, you would pair an unconditioned response (the effect of the drug) with the taking of the pill. In the future, simply taking the pill might evoke the effect of the drug because of conditioning.

But consider two examples. In each of two studies all the patients were diagnosed with duodenal ulcers by endoscopic analysis. Each patient took placebo tablets four times per day for four weeks, after which they were again examined with the endoscope. In each case, we might, as suggested by Dr. Ader, consider this a series of conditioning trials. In one of the studies, done in Germany, twenty-seven of thirty-four placebo-treated patients (79%) were free of ulcers after four weeks (Malchow *et al.* 1978), while in the other study, done in neighboring Denmark under the same circumstances, only five of thirty patients (17%) were better (Gudmand-Hoyer *et al.* 1977). From the point of view of conditioning, the two studies were exactly the same. But the outcome was so different that it is hard to imagine that conditioning had much to do with it. And, of course, none of these patients had taken any of the active drug to "learn" what its effects might be (as happened in Dr. Benedetti's study). Whatever accounts for these differences, it can't logically be what is the *same* in both cases.

Expectations

A number of very imaginative researchers have taken another approach to this issue and speak of placebo effects being the result of "expectancy" or "expectation." Irving Kirsch, the creator of "Trivaricane," the "local anesthetic" discussed in Chapter 2, says that we can account for placebo effects, psychotherapy, hypnosis, and a number of other things, with the concept of "response expectancies." Response expectancies are "anticipations of one's own automatic reactions to various situations and behaviors." So, if you expect that a cup of coffee will wake you up, it will, even if some sneaky researcher has secretly given you decaffeinated coffee (Kirsch and Weixel 1988).

Robert Hahn similarly focuses on the idea of expectation in his definition of "nocebos" which, he says, are "expectations of harmful or painful events that lead to the fulfillment of those expectations" (Hahn 1995:93).

An "expectation" is another way of talking about knowledge or experience. If the doctor tells you that the drug is going to cause terrible side-effects, like headaches or nausea, you are likely to "expect" them. We might, then, attribute your reaction to the medication as a consequence of expectation; or, we might attribute it to your knowledge, obtained from authoritative instruction. But there are many other circumstances where it is plausible to imagine that you know of something in some way, but have no clear sense of it as being "knowledge"; it doesn't form any particular "expectancy." Earlier I described research showing that people who got four placebos per day healed faster than people who only got two a day. Now in the abstract, if we were to ask people "Do you expect that you will get better faster if you take four pills rather than two?" and then gave them two, they might have lower expectations than otherwise. But in the research that was actually done, there was no such prompting. It seems unlikely that, as a general rule, people have any clear expectations at all regarding the instructions "take one with each meal, and one at bedtime" vs. "take one when you get up in the morning, and one at dinner." But people do generally know after the age of three that four means more than two, even if they have never thought carefully (or been instructed) about the significance of this in the context of taking medication. "Knowledge" and "meaning" seem more apt here than does "expectancy."

Similarly, we have seen that Italian men seem to think differently about the color blue than do most other Euro-American men; it is plausible to suggest that this accounts for their unusual reaction to blue sleeping pills. But it seems unlikely that these fans "expect" their fandom to have an effect on their sleep, any more than anyone expects Viagra to work better because it's blue.

The only way we could elicit anything about peoples' expectations on these matters would be to ask them directly, which could plant an expectation that wasn't there before.

In any of these cases – when there are clearly created and measurable expectancies and when there are not – people know things, and experience them meaningfully. They respond to what things mean (whether they "expect" it or not).

11   Ethics, placebos, and meaning

I haven't mentioned it very often, but there are many ethical issues which people routinely raise about placebos. This has been a perennial problem in medicine, I think. The primary problem is that, historically at any rate, when doctors really didn't know what to do for a patient, or simply didn't have any treatment which they thought might be effective, they often gave people inert drugs: bread pills, sugar pills, whatever. In a famous passage from a letter to a physician in 1807, Thomas Jefferson wrote: "One of the most successful physicians I have ever known, has assured me, that he used more bread pills, drops of colored water, & powders of hickory ashes, than of all other medicines put together. It was certainly a pious fraud." Jefferson is forgiving, but he does credit this action to be a "fraud," even if a "pious" one. That the use of placebos seems somehow "fraudulent" is a serious problem for medicine.

The case of the Kwakiutl shaman

One of the great cases, which raises many important issues, can be found in anthropologist Claude Levi-Strauss' famous paper "The Sorcerer and his Magic" (Levi-Strauss 1967b). In it, Levi-Strauss analyzes the case of Quesalid, a Kwakiutl Indian from Vancouver Island in British Columbia, a case originally reported a generation earlier by Franz Boas (Boas 1930). Quesalid had reason to believe that the shamans were cheats and frauds, shamelessly exploiting their patients with trickery. He, tricking the tricksters, managed to get a practicing shaman to take him on as an apprentice. He learned the various techniques of the trade, including the chief trick of the region: "The shaman hides a little tuft of down in the corner of his mouth, and he throws it up, covered with blood, at the proper moment – after having bitten his tongue or made his gums bleed – and solemnly presents it to his patient and the onlookers as the pathological foreign body extracted as a result of his sucking and manipulation" (Levi-Strauss 1967b:169). Having his proof of their trickery, Quesalid was ready to expose them.

But, as part of his training, he was called upon by the family of a sick person and asked to heal the sufferer. He did his trick with the tuft of down, and was stunned to see how successful it was. The patient was healed. He proceeded to have a long and successful career as a shaman, even though he maintained his suspicion of most of his colleagues whom he continued to consider fraudulent. But what about himself? At the end of his story, "we cannot tell, but it is evident that he carries on his craft conscientiously, takes pride in his achievements, and warmly defends the technique of the bloody down against all rival schools. He seems to have completely lost sight of the fallaciousness of the technique which he had so disparaged at the beginning" (Levi-Strauss 1967b:173). Here is a moral dilemma: even if the technique is false, if it helps people, how can he withhold it?

Medicine and deceptions

In a very influential paper published in *Scientific American* in 1974, philosopher Sissela Bok phrased the problem somewhat differently. Writing in the wake of the emergence of the double blind trial as the "gold standard" of medical evidence, Bok argued that deceptive practices, like giving patients inert drugs that they thought were active treatments, was deeply unethical, a form of lying that would be corrosive of medical authority: "Honesty may not be the highest social value; at exceptional times, when survival is at stake, it may have to be set aside. To permit a widespread practice of deception, however, is to set the stage for abuses and growing mistrust" (Bok 1974:23).

In the intervening years, standards have evolved for the use of inert treatments in medical trials which, at least in the United States and Europe, arguably seem to protect patients from the worst abuses. Experiments supported with public funding, say, from the National Institutes of Health, must be approved by a committee at the institution – hospital, university, institute – doing the research. These institutional review boards (usually called IRBs) are ordinarily comprised of a group of professionals – doctors, psychologists, etc. – and others – often ministers, ethicists, etc. – who go over study protocols to see if they satisfactorily protect the participants. Ordinarily, I think these committees do a good job. There are problems, especially with "informed consent." Many people simply can't give informed consent: they may be too sick, too old, or too young (fetuses, infants, small children); they may be mentally handicapped. There are problems with research projects which pay money to participants: on the one hand, it is a lot to ask for people to go to the trouble of participating in an experiment – which would probably involve much more bother than simply being treated for a condition of some sort – without receiving some sort of compensation. However, if the pay is large, it may be, in effect, coercive, forcing someone to participate in a study against his better judgment because he needs money to support his family since he is out of work because he is sick. Such inducements would, of course, have different effects on people of different income levels.

The most disconcerting aspect of informed consent is for someone of sound mind and strong will who is confronting a desperately bad prognosis from an incurable condition. She learns of an experimental procedure which may, or may not, have any effect, and which may be very toxic. How can she decline? Such a decision may be "informed," but it's hard to see it as "consent" if the person thought she simply had no choice, that any chance was better than no chance.

The Declaration of Helsinki

The matter is complicated by a document called the "Declaration of Helsinki," produced by the World Medical Association (World Medical Association 2001). Although the declaration does not carry the force of law, it has significantly influenced many governments and ethical review boards. The latest version of the declaration states that new drugs should only be tested against "the best current treatment" – which has been interpreted by many to mean that placebo controls are only acceptable if there is no effective treatment at all for a condition. The issue here is seen most clearly in the statement that says "in medical research on human subjects, considerations related to the well-being of the human subject should take precedence over the interests of science and society." This has been interpreted by many to suggest that it is unethical, for example, for a pain researcher to organize a study of young people having their wisdom teeth taken out. Since there are effective treatments for such pain, it is wrong to design a study where some portion of those people are given an inert treatment, even if they have volunteered, given informed consent, and there is negligible risk (no more than in the ordinary course of the procedure).

If, for some clearly lethal condition, there were an effective treatment, but researchers had developed a new treatment which was less expensive, or had less toxic side effects, it seems reasonable not to use a placebo treatment group but to compare the new treatment to the old one. Such comparison trials are harder to do than ordinary placebo-controlled trials – they must be larger, require special attention to dropouts, and so on (Temple and Ellenberg 2000; Ellenberg and Temple 2000). In cases, however, where a modest delay in patient treatment with this condition will not cause any serious harm (a new treatment for acne, or PMS, or rheumatoid arthritis, for example) or where the problem is transient (dental surgery pain), it seems reasonable to imagine that consent to participate in experiments can easily be gained in a perfectly satisfactory manner without ethical problems. At least it seems reasonable to me; others strongly disagree.

Placebo mania and placebo phobia

Finally, we must recognize that the whole debate around the issue – one participant has called it "placebo mania" (Rothman 1996) – focuses only on the use of inert medications, "placebos" in the strict sense, and not on the much more complex and interesting issue of "meaning." I can only note that while it may be possible to decide to include, or not to include, a placebo-treated control group in a study, it is simply not possible to decide to include, or not to include, "meaning." It will be there, doing its thing, whether you want it there or not. To ignore *it* seems to me to be the least ethical thing one could possibly do.

Part III

Meaning and human biology

12   The extent (and limits) of meaning

It is clear that what I refer to as the meaning response is far larger and more significant than what happens when people take placebos. Figure 12.1 shows a representation of the relationship between the two situations; they overlap in an important way. Both the placebo effect and the meaning response involve more than simply the reactions of people to inert medications. People taking placebos in an RCT may exhibit regression to the mean (or movement to homeostasis), or bias, or more. Similarly, the physiological or psychological response to meaning – the meaning response – occurs in many more areas than clinical trials.

Sightings

Other authors have extended this net even further than I have. Harvard historian Anne Harrington has described what she calls "sightings,... fauna that live in the same larger territory of human psychobiological functioning in which the placebo effect makes its home as well" (Harrington in press). Among her sightings are these:

- "A room with a view." A study at a suburban Pennsylvanian hospital showed that surgical patients who stayed in a room with a window view of a natural setting got better faster than a matched sample of patients who had a view of a brick wall (Ulrich 1984).
- "Psychosocial dwarfism." A number of studies in the US and Europe have shown that children deprived of a secure bond with a loving care-taker – children in orphanages or abusive situations (even those whose material needs are met) – may grow up physically stunted. They have been shown to have reduced levels of growth hormones. Simply removing them from the situation and providing them with a loving secure home (probably involving people who will talk with them, that is, make life meaningful) can be sufficient to reverse the damage (Mouridsen and Nielsen 1990).
- They "cried until they could not see." Harrington describes the experience of hundreds of Cambodian women "forced by the Khmer Rouge

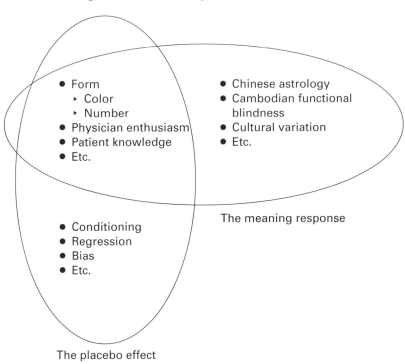

- Form
  - Color
  - Number
- Physician enthusiasm
- Patient knowledge
- Etc.

- Chinese astrology
- Cambodian functional blindness
- Cultural variation
- Etc.

The meaning response

- Conditioning
- Regression
- Bias
- Etc.

The placebo effect

12.1   The meaning response and the placebo effect

to witness the torture and slaughter of those close to them," primarily their husbands and sons. Although there seems to be nothing physically wrong with their eyes, these women are blind; having had to watch such unbearable scenes, they "cried until they could not see" (Drinnan and Marmor 1991; Rozee and Van Boemel 1989).

It is clear, from this perspective, that the placebo effect in the strict sense is only a special case of the meaning response. But it is also a particularly interesting one, since it is subject to experimentation which would simply be impossible in these other situations. One cannot randomize a group of people so that half end up being Chinese and the other half Anglo-American; one can't randomize people to being Cambodian refugees, or to experiencing grotesque suffering. But one can randomize people to get blue or red pills, or to get shots rather than pills. That is, in the case of medications, it is both ethically and practically possible to experiment with these issues. Unfortunately, with some very special exceptions – work by Levine, Fields, Gracely, and Benedetti, for example – most of the work which we *can* draw on to understand these issues has not been done explicitly to learn about the role of meaning in medicine, but as a contingent element of other investigations in pharmacology or physiology.

Given the possibility that there is such a wide range of similar phenomena – where biology is so fully engaged with experience, culture, and meaning – why is it that these matters are so often neglected, rejected, or despised?

The land of Oz

As an example of this rejection, it is worth noting the extraordinary buzz which was generated by an article about the placebo effect which appeared in the spring of 2001. Using a meta-analysis of medical trials which had three arms – treatment group, placebo group, and untreated group – the authors argued that there were no differences between outcomes in placebo-treated and untreated groups. Conceding that the studies of pain which they reviewed did show an effect in the placebo-treated groups, they concluded nonetheless that there was "little evidence in general that placebos had powerful clinical effects," and that there was "no justification for the use of placebos" (Hróbjartsson and Gøtzsche 2001). An editorial accompanied the paper and compared placebos to the Wizard of Oz, "who was powerful because others thought he was powerful" (Bailar 2001).

The study was an odd one. It compared studies from a huge range of conditions including hypertension and herpes infection, which was reasonable enough. But it also included studies of alcohol abuse, smoking, obesity, common cold, phobia, schizophrenia, orgasmic difficulties, Alzheimer's disease, faecal soiling, and marital discord. "Marital discord" – what medical treatment is there for marital discord? Indeed, many of the items listed have no obvious medical treatment and are not really treatable at all: there is no cure for schizophrenia or Alzheimer's disease. My hunch at the time was that, if the authors had collected the results of the active treatment groups in these studies, they too would have been no more effective than the no-treatment groups (but they didn't collect those data). Indeed, it is interesting to imagine what sorts of conditions might receive approval for a no-treatment group in the first place. It would be quite difficult to get approval to withhold treatment from a group of seriously ill patients if an effective treatment were available. We have already noted, for example, that angina is a serious condition which displays large meaning responses; but there are effective treatments for angina, and it is hard to imagine that a study could be approved which withheld treatment from such patients. Indeed, there were no studies of angina in the meta-analysis. And, of course, we have already noted the conceptual and practical problems of creating a no-treatment group in the first place – remember "medicine by binoculars." Evaluating, diagnosing, and admitting patients to a study, and then following their medical progress, is not "nothing," and is not "inert."

In sum, I was less than impressed with the study. But apparently I was the only one! The paper got enormous press coverage, on the front page of the *New York Times* and in the *Washington Post, The Los Angeles Times*, and an enormous number of other newspapers. It was on National Public Radio, and featured in *Newsweek* and *Time*. It was everywhere. A cartoon in *Time* used the study as a sort of metaphor for modern times, saying that "the recent stock market boom was fueled by the placebo effect" and showing a woman thinking "Subscribing to this cell-phone service makes me feel like I'm striking a blow against conformity!" It was really pretty funny. Less funny was Ellen Goodman, normally a very sensible columnist for the *Boston Globe*, who wrote that the placebo effect "carries the harsh sound of a quack. It's a scam, and when properly labeled nobody buys it" (Goodman 2001). One of the most powerful forces in our lives – the biological consequences of social, human, and meaningful interaction – had been tossed into the ash can.

Placebo socket wrenches and Dodge trucks

Why? Why is it so easy to reject a set of ideas which allow us to approach and understand such a rich, diverse set of phenomena from Pennebaker's disclosure theory to Benedetti's placebo analgesia, from menopause to blind Cambodians? A few weeks after the study – and press storm – appeared, a group of Canadian researchers published a fascinating account of their work with brain scans which indicated that, in patients with Parkinson's disease, placebo treatment actually caused the release of dopamine (the loss of cells which produce dopamine is essentially the cause of Parkinson's) (de La Fuente-Fernandez *et al.* 2001). It is conceivable that meaningful intervention could bring relief for people with this terrible disease. But there were no editorials in *Science*, where the paper was published, and no front page stories in the *Times* or the *Post*, and no cartoons in *Time*. Why?

In part, I think, this is because there is no useful theory to guide investigation and to suggest interesting experiments. These phenomena, especially placebo effects, seem to most people to be "simply psychological": "The mind," people say, "tells the body what to do." This accounts, perhaps, for the single most consistent effort over the years to account for placebo phenomena, the search for the characteristics of the "placebo reactor" (who will be dependent, or authoritative, or the like). This research, as we saw in Chapter 4, was fruitless and led nowhere. But the theory which underlies it seems to remain. (One wonders which ears the body uses to listen to what the mind is saying.)

There is another quality of this situation which is hard to specify, but which I think I can explain. Having thought and written about these issues for a long time, I can attest to the reactions that people have to serious discussions of the placebo effect. It is rare to find someone who, on learning of some aspect of this issue, doesn't say something like "Man, this stuff is really weird," or "It's just amazing how this happens; I mean, it's really hard to believe." Even physicians who experience this phenomenon every day express similar kinds of surprise, sometimes tinged with anger. "So, when *you're* sick, do you want me to treat you with [sneer] *placebos?*" Minimally, meaning responses seem very surprising to people, perhaps especially to physicians. Why?

I would suggest that contemporary, Western culture has a highly mechanistic view of the way the world works. Our sense of the universe is very Newtonian in its nature: energy is conserved, only one thing can be in a space at a time; falling bodies fall, and billiard balls bounce the way geometry says they should. And human beings are made up of bodies with minds in them; and the mind is in the head (not the leg or chest), sort of a computer. Before computers were commonplace, people thought of the head as containing something like a steam engine, or a complicated clock – whatever was the most clever technology of the day. It's a very mechanical perspective, and has been for centuries.

Consider a thought experiment: we fabricate some placebo socket wrenches. They look like socket wrenches, sound like them, feel like them. But we design them so that when you put the socket over the loose nut and tighten it, the nut will stay loose. We secretly place these wrenches in the tool boxes of a randomly selected set of mechanics at the car repair shop. Now, if we discovered that the nuts these mechanics were working on really *did* tighten up, we would have good reason to be surprised. The only thing that can tighten up nuts is a (real) wrench.

Many people see the human body as a machine, rather like a Dodge truck. If the body is a machine, then we might well be surprised each time we find people responding to inert medications, as, in our thought experiment, lug nuts responded to an inert wrench. People *are* surprised; so I conclude that they think of people as machines. Working with a similar metaphor, one student of these matters put it this way: "In the mechanistic tradition that still underlies much of modern biomedicine, believing in the power of a placebo to erase pain is as irrational as filling the gas tank of your car with Earl Grey tea" (Morris 1997).

Recently there has been a whole spate of talk about the hardware and software of the brain; and, conversely, people talk about machines having "intelligence." Of course there are things about animals and humans which are like machines: certain physical principles of levers, pulleys, fluid mechanics, and the like, are common to both; there are many complex chemical processes that can occur in the body and in a test tube, and so on. One of the greatest analytic mistakes a person can make, however, is to let substantial similarities obscure fundamental differences (keep the story of the Trojan horse in mind).

People are not machines. People are far more complex than any machine. We have, in this book, spent a lot of time addressing "pain." But we have considered only a fraction of the complexity of pain and its regulation. We have considered the endogenous opiates (the endorphins) and their role in pain control. But I have not indicated anything of the other actions of the endorphins in the body: they play important roles throughout the entire organism, affecting everything from respiration to urination, from eating to exercising, from the immune system to the heart. A review of research on endogenous opiates published in the year 1999 was 60 pages long and had 603 references – all for 1999 (Vaccarino and Kastin 2000)![31] This complexity simply cannot be reduced to the notion "the mind tells the body what to do."

Independent and dependent variables

The primacy of the mechanical shows itself in another way, even in the work of the most imaginative and creative researchers. Typically, in mechanics or physics, one is interested in the relationship between two variables. Suppose one wants to see the relation between x and y, between, say, calories ingested and weight. Our theory would most likely be that the more calories someone consumed, the more he or she would weigh; that is, calorie consumption would somehow "cause" weight, or, weight is a function of calories. And we would be likely to make a graph, putting

---

[31] Here is the abstract of the paper, just to give you the flavor of the thing: "This paper is the twenty-second installment of the annual review of research concerning the opiate system. It summarizes papers published during 1999 that studied the behavioral effects of the opiate peptides and antagonists, excluding the purely analgesic effects, although stress-induced analgesia is included. The specific topics covered this year include stress; tolerance and dependence; learning, memory, and reward; eating and drinking; alcohol and other drugs of abuse; sexual activity, pregnancy, and development; mental illness and mood; seizures and other neurologic disorders; electrical-related activity; general activity and locomotion; gastrointestinal, renal, and hepatic function; cardiovascular responses; respiration and thermoregulation; and immunologic responses."

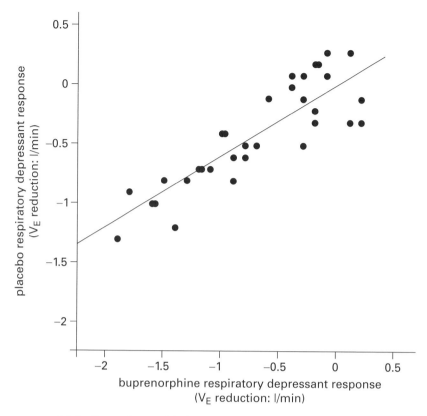

12.2   Dependent and independent variables. The figures shows the relationship between changes in respiration – in V, the "minute volume,"
the number of liters of air breathed per minute – following an opiate
injection (on the x, or horizontal, axis) and changes in the respiration
following an injection of inert saline solution (on the y, or vertical axis).
(*Source*: Benedetti *et al.* 1998)

calories consumed on the horizontal axis, the "x-axis", and the weight on
the vertical axis, the "y-axis." In standard parlance, the x-axis is where
we map the "independent variable," while the y-axis is where we map the
"dependent variable." Figure 12.2 demonstrates this from an important
paper by Fabrizio Benedetti. The graph shows the change in respiration
following an injection of an opiate (buprenorphine) or a placebo; each
point on the graph shows the results for the drug, and for the placebo,
for one individual. The key here is not the data itself (interesting as they
are), but the structure of the data, the way they are displayed, which,

in the standard argot, has the response to *the drug* as the independent variable, on the x-axis, and the response to *placebo* as the dependent variable, on the y-axis. But as we have seen, opiates activate an endogenous pain control system (and, in the process, suppress respiration); the opiate, mimicking the endorphins, acts to augment a primary, or independent, system in a secondary way. It seems far more plausible to reverse the axes on this graph, to show the placebo responses as the independent variables and the drug responses as the dependent variables; individuals with endogenous opiate systems highly sensitive to activation with language and meaning are also highly sensitive to opiates. In general, the drug process piggybacks on the internal, endogenous process, and is a function of it.

It seems sensible to propose as a hypothesis that this is true in other circumstances as well. In ulcer disease, there are clearly two ways to facilitate the healing of ulcers. First of all, it is worth mentioning that many ulcers ultimately will heal themselves with no intervention at all; it is not at all clear how this might happen, but something is going on in there! It is also clear that there are two quite different kinds of treatments which can heal ulcers (that is, heal them faster than they might otherwise heal by themselves). First, there are many very effective "hydrogen blockers," drugs which inhibit the production of hydrogen, hence limiting the production of acid (HCL); it is not clear how this helps, but perhaps in the acid-reduced environment, the mucous layer of the stomach can more easily cover over the ulcer. Second, ulcers can be healed with antibiotics. Ulcers are associated with bacteria called *Helicobacter pylori*. By eliminating this bacteria with a very potent antibiotic treatment, the ulcers will be eliminated.[32]

So, when ulcers get better after people have taken placebos, what happened? No one knows. But it certainly seems plausible to imagine that two possibilities exist. First, the amount of acid might be reduced somehow; or second, the immune system may activate to eliminate the bacterial infection. No one knows if either one of these two factors is involved. But no one has ever looked, either. Neither of these possibilities seems reasonable in a certain (mechanical) sense, in the sense of the placebo socket wrench, or Earl Grey gasoline. And, of course, these are not mutually exclusive; they may both occur, and, indeed, there may be a third or fourth factor. As noted, ulcers do seem to go away by themselves sometimes. That is to say, there are endogenous mechanisms which act to heal these lesions; it is plausible to suggest that meaningful experiences may be able to activate these processes, whatever they may be.

---

[32] I don't say that the bacteria "cause" ulcers because many people (in fact most people) have them in their gut, but do not have ulcers.

But the general idea is that, at least some of the time, it seems reasonable to understand that drugs activate some sort of existing biological process which facilitates healing. And it is also possible that, at least some of the time, meaningful experiences might activate these same existing biological processes.

Some well-known drugs do *not* do this. Aspirin, and the rest of the non-steroidal anti-inflammatory drugs (NSAIDs), seem not to work this way. Unlike morphine, which *activates* a pain *control* system, the NSAIDs do the reverse. They *inhibit* a system which (among other things) *causes* pain. As noted earlier in Chapter 8, this system involves a class of hormone-like chemicals known as prostaglandins. Prostaglandins are produced by an enzyme known as cyclooxygenase (COX). NSAIDs inhibit COX, and, thereby, the production of prostaglandins. The prostaglandins are very important chemicals which are involved in the pain response, in the development of inflammatory responses (important in wound healing), and in temperature regulation. They also are crucial in the process whereby you maintain the mucous layer in your gut. Taking an aspirin can, then, reduce pain and fever; but this can lead to irritation of the stomach, and, in large doses, can lead to ulcers. Since fever is actually part of the immune response – fever enhances the body's response to infection – taking aspirin to reduce fever or the aches and pains of a cold or virus can actually lengthen the illness, and can marginally lengthen the time that someone else can catch your cold (Pittman, Veale, and Cooper 1976; Graham *et al.* 1990); it may make you feel better, but your cold might last longer. I know of no evidence to suggest that the effect of aspirin can be induced in the body as a meaning response. In several experiments when there were meaning responses evident in people given NSAIDS, they were reversible with naloxone. Naloxone is an "opiate antagonist," not an "aspirin antagonist."

A general theory

A general theory then might go something like this. There are several sorts of neurological processes: those which are, and those which are not, sensitive to "external" stimuli; and among the latter, those which involve "conscious" or "cognitive" responses and those which don't (Table 12.1). Some things (Type I) just "go on by themselves," responding primarily to internal matters. These include such things as transferring oxygen to the tissues and transferring carbon dioxide to the blood, processing blood in the spleen, accumulating urine, maintaining the mucous lining of the gut, and so on. These autonomous processes are all under some form of central neurological and/or endocrine control, and they are by and large

Table 12.1. *Types of neurological control*

Type I	Insensitive to external influence		1. Nourishment absorbed from the gut 2. Gas balance in the blood 3. Peristalsis
Type II	Sensitive to external influence	Not conscious or cognitive	4. Hearing, seeing, tasting 5. Hand-eye coordination 6. Pain
Type III		Conscious or cognitive	7. Language 8. Classification 9. Intention

out of human conscious or deliberate control. They are not, of course, insulated from experience, but the connection to it is mediated by other neurological processes, particularly emotional ones. For example, the classic signs of acute stress – a "fight or flight reaction" caused by fear or panic – include significant increases in heart rate and blood pressure, decrease in activity of the gut (digestion can be taken care of later), and significant alterations of the activity of the immune system. That these alterations are a response to the *emotions*, not the experience that generated the emotions, is evident in modern stress diseases which are due not to *acute* stress (from chasing prey, or being chased) but to *chronic* stress (from constant demands of school or work). These functions respond primarily to internal physiological and psychological states.

Some neurological processes (Type II) are clearly affected by external events which are experienced, but not consciously. The ordinary five "senses" are good examples of this: the whole point of a "sense" is that it processes external stimuli and makes judgments of some sort, or leads to a response of some sort. As you walk up a set of stairs, you characteristically watch the steps, but you take no conscious control of the muscles in your arm and hand (on the banister), or of your back or legs, or of your balance. You decide to "walk up the stairs," and several dozen muscles, under various sorts of regulation by your nervous system, do their things, and there you are on the second floor. If you try this with a blindfold on, you will get a sense of how much external information is needed to do the task easily. Probably you will still be able to "feel" your way up the stairs, but it will involve different senses, and certainly you will do it less comfortably (and more "consciously"). Other similar situations might include things like "this is bitter, spit it out", or "that's hot, my hand springs away from the iron." There is some evidence that with biofeedback training, some control can be exerted over some of these, but only very little, and not very reliably; one study, for example, shows only trivial amounts of control can be developed over finger temperature (Kewman and Roberts 1980). And even though these types of stimuli might not be cognitive or conscious in the ordinary senses of those terms, they might involve meaningful events on occasion: the notion, for example, that you might get hungry an hour after eating a big dinner in a Chinese restaurant involves the scrambling of certain kinds of meaning of which you are ordinarily (but not necessarily) unaware.

Finally, there are those stimuli (Type III) which involve consciousness, choice, decision making, ritual, etc.: the neurological processes which characteristically make us human. These processes let us know there is a difference between the words "John hit Bill" and "Bill hit John," however those ideas might be expressed in a thousand different languages. While many of these might seem to have little effect on neurological states, we know that there are many that are very important. You can sit in a quiet corner, in a comfortable chair reading a Stephen King novel and be terrified: your heart is racing, you are breathing hard, and you could lose control of your bladder; all that and more as you interpret little black marks on a page. And we know that if someone in a white coat with a stethoscope in the pocket tells you that she is about to give you "an injection of a powerful pain killer," often enough, an injection of inert, sterile saline solution will stop your pain.

Of course, everything is related. If you have a terrible argument with your boyfriend while you are eating lunch (Type III activity), it might influence the absorption of nutrition from the gut (Type I). And, if you have some sort of gastrointestinal disorder, a real pain in the gut (Type I), you might find yourself grumpy and argumentative (Type III). So these things are only conceptually distinct.

Regardless of the fact that these distinctions are conceptual, meaning responses would ordinarily be of Type III. There is some evidence which suggests that the musical and rhythmic elements found in many healing and other religious ceremonies around the world can affect certain brain wave patterns; these things can apparently alter consciousness in various ways, inducing trance states, for example, which might be something like hypnosis. One recent study has shown that relaxing music reduced heart rate, respiratory rate, and the amount of oxygen the heart used in patients who had just suffered heart attacks; the people who listened to the music fared better than a group of similar patients who were simply placed in a quiet, restful room, and better than the "ordinary care group" (White 1999). This would be a "Type II" intervention.

The key idea here is that meaning responses or placebo effects (in the strict sense) have to involve physiological mechanisms which can be influenced from "outside." An important example is the immune system which is clearly influenced by perceptions, experiences, and emotions; the immune system might be seen as having aspects of all three types in Table 12.1 – it responds to internal and external matters. Indeed, one researcher suggested years ago that the immune system should be regarded as an additional sensory organ (Blalock 1984). Roger Booth and his colleagues have suggested in a number of ways that "meaning" in the psycho-socio-cultural sense relates to the *self*, which the immune system differentiates from *non-self*, while maintaining a coherent relationship between the self and the context within which it exists (Booth and Ashbridge 1993). Andrew Watkins has described perceptions, emotions, and immunity as "an integrated homoeostasis" (Watkins 1995). From this perspective, it seems more likely that meaning responses will be effective when they are aimed at the immune system than when aimed at the prostaglandin system.

If this notion can be shown to be wrong – that is, if the prostaglandin system *can* be influenced somehow meaningfully – all the better. We learn something either way. One significant advantage of this approach is that it readily suggests many testable hypotheses.

When meaning responses don't occur

In this book I have tried to describe the thoroughgoing way that meaningful processes can influence human health for better or for worse. It is quite clear that these things can and do happen, and that they form a very significant portion of the whole range of effects of any medical system, conventional or alternative, Western or otherwise. And the effects can be profound.

So, why is it that these effects – often highly desirable – occur so erratically? Why don't they happen to everyone all the time?

Figure 12.3 reminds us how much variation there is in conventional medical outcomes. The left graph, showing drug group variations in 117 trials ranging from 40% healing to 100% healing, and the right graph, showing placebo group healing ranging from 0% to 100%, indicate just how broadly these things can vary; nothing happens to everybody all the time (well, almost nothing). Why? In this particular case, there are a number of possibilities: varying portions of these individuals may have gotten better without treatment; there may be different strains of bacteria involved; there may be national or other cultural factors involved; etc. But the same kinds of variations occur in much more tightly controlled studies, lacking the possibilities of different strains of bacteria, or cultural factors, and so on. There is no clear theory to go on here.

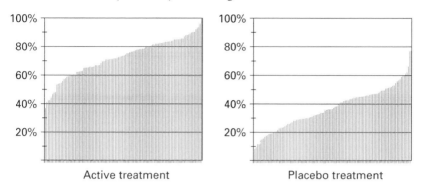

12.3   Variability in outcome of active and placebo treatment for ulcer disease. Four-week healing rates for active and placebo treatment in 117 trials of hydrogen blockers for ulcer disease.

One possibility has been proposed by Dr. Nick Humphrey, an evolutionary psychologist from the London School of Economics. He argues that, from an evolutionary perspective, one has to recognize that some of these healing processes are not "free," and they are not without risk. Evidence exists, he says, to show that various stresses in an animal's life – like cold temperatures of winter, reproductive activities (producing breeding colors in birds, for example), infant care, or internal parasites – can suppress the activity of the immune system (see, for example, Sheldon and Verhulst 1996; Svensson *et al.* 1998). There are times, Humphrey argues, when it is more reasonable for an individual to continue being sick, and not expend the resources necessary to get well, since those resources may be needed later, perhaps for other, more serious problems:

The human capacity for responding to placebos [we would, of course, say 'meaning'] is in fact not necessarily adaptive in its own right (indeed it can sometimes even be maladaptive). Instead, this capacity is an emergent property of something else that *is* genuinely adaptive: namely, a specially designed procedure for 'economic resource management' that is . . . one of the key features of the 'natural health-care service' which has evolved in ourselves and other animals to help us deal throughout our lives with repeated bouts of sickness, injury, and other threats to our well-being. (Humphrey 2002)

The British professor Humphrey makes a rather lighthearted analogy with the British National Health Service, and compares the rational allocation policies of that institution with the ways in which individual persons or other animals "allocate" their energetic and other resources. He notes that there are times when it really makes sense to delay relieving symptoms of illness or injury. Pain, for example, has the effect of making us "lie low" for a time while an injury (a sprained ankle, for example) heals. Taking a drug to relieve that pain, or responding to a placebo injection, might allow you to walk on the ankle before you really should, which might prolong the healing period. Likewise, he notes that the fever which accompanies a cold or influenza works much like pain, making us feel badly, so we conserve our strength; moreover, a raised body temperature leads to a shorter period of infection as the increased heat apparently acts to reduce the viability of the infectious agent (Graham *et al.* 1990).

Dr. Humphrey also notes that the same symptom or experience can have very different significance in different circumstances. Consider pain: suppose you sprain your ankle while you are chasing a gazelle "and the pain has made you stop – then . . . [the pain is] going to save your ankle from further damage even if it means your losing the gazelle. But suppose you yourself are being chased by a lion – then if you stop it will likely be the end of you."

His argument is more complex than this, and more interesting. It is also highly speculative, and contains a fair number of "just so stories" (and lots of [very hypothetical] running from lions). It does, however, provide a framework for thinking about these issues.

13 Conclusions: many claims, many issues

I have made many claims in this book. Some of them are quite straightforward, while others are more anomalous. Some have lots of good evidence, while some have less. Some issues seem clearly nailed down, while for others I have said that "more research is needed." Now I want to summarize the whole picture of the meaning response, and indicate what we need to know most to make this powerful human process more understandable, and maybe even more useful.

People live in rich and complex worlds of their own construction. Whether they are nuclear physicists, Jesuit priests, or members of the Taliban in Afghanistan; British, French or German; Navajo, Seneca, or Maya; in any case, people view the same world in many different ways, making sense of it, making it meaningful in many different ways. It is easy to overstate the case for cultural differences: all societies have families, provide food, speak languages, and share understandings. But the differences remain profound; I would argue, for example, that these differences are far greater and far more important than any genetic variations among human beings. What might appear to an outside observer to be very minuscule differences (e.g., that the bread and wine "are" the body and blood of Christ rather than that the bread and wine "represent" the body and blood of Christ) can be matters of enormous importance (the issue of "transubstantiation" was – indeed still is – probably the most important theological issue in the many disputes of the Protestant Reformation).

It is quite clear that these matters of understanding and belief, fully and fundamentally shaped by and reflected in language, make the world seem to be very different to different people. The Russian language simply has no word which means the same thing as the English word "mind." The closest thing, the one translators usually select, is *duša*, which much more closely approximates the English word "soul." "Thoughts related to *duša* can hardly be thought in ordinary (idiomatic) English, and since in Russian a very high proportion of thoughts seem to be linked with the concept of *duša*, to a Russian the universe of Anglo-Saxon culture

seems to be characterized by *bezdušie*, lack of *duša*, . . . 'soul-less-ness' "
(Wierzbicka 1989:55).

It may be worth noting that few languages have a word which easily accommodates the English word "mind." In my little pocket French/English dictionary, the first translation for "mind" is *esprit*. But looking up "esprit," we find these English choices: "spirit, ghost, soul, mind, wit." "Mind" comes fourth. Descartes, in his famous work which differentiated what we call in English "mind and body", actually wrote of *âme* and *corps*. No problem with "corps," or body, but *âme* hasn't much to do with English "mind"; my little dictionary suggests "soul, spirit, core, heart, life." No "mind" at all. In my German dictionary, for "mind" we get "Gemüt, Geist, Neigung, Absicht." The first suggestions in the same dictionary for translating each of those words into English are, respectively, "disposition," "spirit," "inclination," and "intention." The word Freud used in German, inevitably translated into English as "mind," was "die Seele," or "soul."

Wierzbicka concludes that such lexical differences "can be regarded as clues to the different cultural universes associated with different languages." This is the case even among cultures as similar as these – American, British, French, German, Russian – which have shared populations, languages, monarchies, literacy, and education for a millennium, and, more recently, science. Regardless of their shared histories, their different languages – aspects of different cultures – engage different cultural universes. To some important degree, we live in different universes.

These rich and different worlds are primarily different because of "meaning." What does it mean to say that "something means something?" Obviously a knotty problem. Meaning is a relationship between two things. Such meanings can be of many types; here I will describe three. A dark cloud means rainstorm. This is a metonymic sort of meaning where a part of a thing represents the whole; the cloud is part of the rainstorm it represents (as we have seen in "counting noses" or "military brass"). A statue of a man on a horse is somewhat different, an *iconic* representation: the man and horse represented are not part of the statue. The statue, in this case, shares the form of ("looks like") the thing represented. In the case of, say, a Hindu "lingam" or of a Greek milemarker of the type known as a "herm"– named after the god Hermes, the traveler and thief (Brown 1969) – the relationship may be less obviously representational; both lingam and herm are "phallic symbols" which share the form of the, well, the thing represented (similarly, the shape of the monument representing the man Americans call "the Father of our Country" in Washington, DC, seems to be no accident). A third type of meaning occurs in symbolic language where the relationship between the sign and the thing represented, between the word "cat" and the furry quadruped, is arbitrary. "Cat" isn't part of the cat, doesn't look like the cat, and isn't shaped like any part of the cat. One of the most powerful qualities to such symbols is that one can use them without having the thing represented (the thing it "means") in the room at all. This means, too, that one can talk about things which have no material referents at all, like "mind," "Seele," "duša," or "âme"; it may be worth noting that, easy as they are to talk about, it is much harder to find a way to make a statue of "mind" or "duša" than of a general or a horse.

In all these different sorts of representations, meaning is a relationship, a correspondence between one thing and another, literal or otherwise. Knowing how these kinds of relationships work – being able, in the famous example from Clifford Geertz, to tell the difference between a "twitch and a wink" (Geertz 1973) – is a hallmark of humanity.

These kinds of meanings are important parts of human thinking, but they also affect life itself very powerfully. Moreover, meaning affects biology (life); biology (life) is meaningful. If someone tells you a risque joke, a story about something that never happened, you may "blush." If you see a picture of a luscious plate of food (A + 2b), your mouth might water (you might begin to salivate). If someone tells you this pill is a powerful pain killer, and you take it, it might induce you to start producing endogenous opiates and reduce your pain. Meaning affects life.

The reverse is also true: for example, in most places in the world, sex is very meaningful. Attaching meaning to sexual difference creates gender. "Gender roles" are among the most powerful and influential forces in our world, like it or not. The same obviously is true for trivial biological differences such as skin color and epicanthic folds, which often assume meaning far beyond any biological importance they may have. Young people are aware of just how meaningful other minor biological phenomena can be: pimples, or a mole on the nose, or breasts which are "too big" or "too small," can cause enormous amounts of grief for people not because they are biologically significant, but because they are meaningful. In a searing book, *Illness as Metaphor*, writer (and breast cancer survivor) Susan Sontag described how two diseases in particular – tuberculosis and cancer – have been used as metaphors for a vast range of negative experiences, which then add to the burden of the people who experience these diseases (Sontag 1977). If someone with cancer reads that some "bad" thing ("Communism," a "spy," a "scandal") is "a cancer within," it's hard to imagine how this could make you feel good. A decade later, Sontag wrote a book titled *AIDS and Its Metaphors*, again noting the devastating effects of the meanings which we attribute to diseases on the people who experience them (Sontag 1988). In both these books, she urges us simply to stop using such medical metaphors. Urging human beings to stop attributing meaning to phenomena is as plausible as urging us to stop breathing. But I understand her sentiment; you will too, if you read her books. Meaning affects life; Life affects meaning.

Given that biology is meaningful, and meaning is biological, and recognizing that meaning can vary dramatically from one place to another, it ought not be surprising that biology is local, that the "same" biological processes in different places have different "effects" on people. Clearly there are limits here: we are all mortal regardless of culture; we all need oxygen in our tissues; and we all need to consume and digest food, to sleep, to dream. But much is also biologically flexible. Our examples earlier involved the varying experience of menopause around the world, and the effects of astrological understandings on the health of Chinese-Americans. A very controversial example involves the relationship between "depression" and "somatization." People with psychiatric illnesses like depression are said to have two sorts of symptoms, either "psychological" symptoms (like worries, fears, sadness, feelings of regret, guilt, suicidal ideas, panic, and so on) or "somatic" symptoms (like pain or "chronic pain," headaches, chest pains, difficulty breathing, skin rashes, irritable bowels, and so on). Some develop psychological (or "mental") symptoms, while others develop somatic (or "physical") symptoms. A widespread approach to these different symptoms suggests that somatic symptoms of distress are more common among people of various non-Western cultures – particularly from Africa and Asia – and that psychological symptoms are more common in the West (Gaw 1993). A recent review of the subject has suggested that this is far too simplistic a view and, in particular, that somatic symptoms of psychological distress are universal (Kirmayer and Young 1998). The authors note that a long attention to, and disparagement of, somatic symptoms is a result of Western dualistic thinking which sees mind and body as fundamentally separate entities (recall our discussion of the ambiguity – for English speakers – of the concept of "mind" in the first place!) and represent a cultural construction of disease, its meaning and value, in the west. Western "patients who complain of somatic symptoms in the absence of physiological confirmation [as happens with Gulf War Syndrome, chronic fatigue syndrome, and the like] are then suspect." But Kirmayer and Young also note that other medical traditions, like the Indian Ayurveda and Chinese traditional medicine, did not make bold distinctions between "mental" and "physical" illnesses (perhaps because they don't distinguish so clearly between "mind" and body in the first place). So there is less reason in these other traditions to stigmatize physical symptoms of emotional distress. In any case, conditions as different as menopause, chronic pain, cancer, and depression are experienced differently as their meanings and moral valences shift from one culture to another. Biology is, to some degree, local.

In particular, even after factoring out confounding variables, psychiatric talk therapies of all types are extremely helpful to many people for many conditions the world around. We have seen that all forms of psychotherapy are helpful. As people create stories from their lives, restructure the flow of life into meaningful objects, they are able to relieve much distress, suffering, and many physical problems; people using psychotherapy are better than 75% of people with similar problems who don't do it. Moreover, we have seen from Dr. Pennebaker's work that it doesn't take much to do this: writing for ten or fifteen minutes about traumatic experience three or four times can have a dramatic positive effect on long-term health, as can simply assessing your own general level of health as "excellent."

In particular, people can respond to inert pills or injections. We have seen this in many areas of medicine as people have experienced ulcer healing, pain relief (especially for headaches with brand name placebos), reduced blood pressure, and a range of other phenomena. Recall that the one thing we can be utterly certain of is that these changes are *not* due to placebos; placebos are inert and, therefore, don't "do" anything. But they *can be* meaningful. This meaning can activate biological processes, and it can enhance the effectiveness of powerful drugs like morphine.

Moreover, people can respond to sham surgery. We have considered sham surgery for several conditions – for heart disease, arthritis, Ménière's disease, and so on. This often seems particularly striking and magical (or problematic and dangerous) to observers. Surgery, after all, is typically a mechanical intervention in the body. It seems "natural" to set broken limbs or remove bad teeth (even chimpanzees do it). Surgery is done for logical reasons; if something is broken, fix it. So it seems particularly anomalous to us that even though something wasn't really fixed (with sham surgery), it got better nonetheless. It sounds like what might happen at a dishonest car repair shop where you are assured that they replaced the brake shoes, but they didn't. The remarkable thing is that, as we have seen, even when the laser was never turned on, or the artery never ligated (or the brake pads not replaced), large numbers of heart patients got much better anyway (and the car stops; well, it might if it were a person).

These responses occur also when people are given active medication, or "real" surgery. This is one of the hardest things to demonstrate, and it is one of the most difficult elements to make convincing, especially for clinicians, who are often mystified by the fact of their pills. The magic dust in their eyes blinds them to the many factors underlying human healing, including meaning along with autonomous healing, regression to the mean, conditioning, and all the other things that might play a role one time or another.

The effect of meaning is a human universal. Although the evidence is only inferential, it seems likely that this is very common across space and time, in all cultures since the dawn of language. All cultures known have some sort of medical system. Nowhere do people leave their friends, family, or neighbors to their own devices when they are sick, injured, or distressed. One of the first Neanderthal fossils discovered around the turn of the twentieth century at La Chapelle aux Saintes, in France, had substantial arthritis in his spine (see Figure 13.1). He had lost all of his molars and half of his premolars. His jaw had long since healed from the loss of all those teeth, indicating that he had lived a long time in this diminished condition. It is unlikely that he was doing a lot of hunting of wild beasts with Mousterian tools; his friends and family were probably caring for him and feeding him.

Another middle Paleolithic fossil from Shanidar, a famous cave site in Iraq occupied roughly 60,000 years ago, is of an individual who somehow lost his left forearm. His wound healed, and he lived for many years with one arm. Moreover, according to C. Loring Brace, who has closely examined the fossil remains, "he had taken a fearsome whack on the left front side of his head and lost the sight of his left eye. It may have affected his motor control of his right side. There are sprains and arthritic signs in his right leg, and his right 5th metatarsal [footbone] had been broken. With only one eye, missing his right lower arm, and with problems in his right leg, he certainly needed help surviving." Also from Shanidar there is evidence of the use of medicinal plants over 60,000 years ago; pollen and actual flower remains from half a dozen medicinal plants (yarrow, blue cornflower, grape hyacinths, joint fir, and hollyhock) were found in a burial in the cave (Solecki 1975; Leroi-Gourhan 1975; Leroi-Gourhan 1998).

Around the world, native peoples always have a system of medicine, often two systems. The first is usually a rather informal familial medicine, similar to what most of us would use for everyday cuts and bruises, colds and indispositions. The second is usually a rather more formal system, often with fairly elaborate symbolic elements, as seen in those societies which have developed shamans and other medical professionals like, for example, the famous singers of the Navajo. In each case, it is common for people to use a broad range of medicinal plants, many of which include very useful drugs (like opium in poppies, the salicylates ["natural aspirin"] found in willows, birches and wintergreen, quinine in Cinchona,

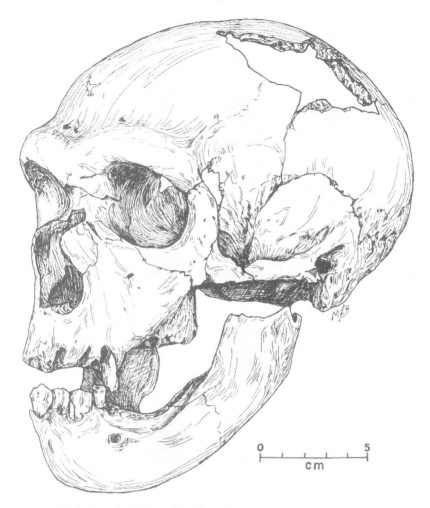

13.1   The Old Man of La Chapelle. The incisors were lost after death, but the molars and premolars were lost long before he died, as can be seen from the fact that the jaw and mandible have completely healed. (*Source*: Brace, Nelson, and Korn 1971:83)

etc.) (Moerman 1998b). In all these places, medicines are understood to be meaningful and important; often they exist within a rich religious and mythical tradition which explains the plant's action, often in terms of its physical appearance. It is probably the case that the meaning attached to these medicines is far more explicit and vivid than are the meanings in Western medicine, which are much more implicit (big pills are powerful;

blue pills are sedatives). For example, among the most important and powerful medicinal plants used by the Iroquois are those known to grow on graves (Herrick 1978; Herrick and Snow 1995).

But, as I noted earlier in my discussion of Navajo medicine in Chapter 3, while it is plausible to believe that these meanings have effects similar to those associated with Western drugs, doctors, hospitals, and so on, there is really very little evidence to show that it is the case since there simply is no research on which to base such a claim, and such research would be very hard to design if you *were* to do it. What "inert" action would you select to compare to a shaman's trance or a Navajo song cycle? It is hard enough to compare such things in many areas of Western medicine (especially surgery) as well as among Western nations; it is practically impossible to do so beyond that range. Nonetheless, it seems reasonable to assume that these processes are universally part of the human commitment to help one another get better.

Certain biological systems of great evolutionary age are probably the mechanisms responsible for much of the meaning response. These include the immune system, the endogenous opiates, the "stress hormones" (adrenaline, epinephrine), etc. – important elements in the way organisms mediate the environment are (unlike many other neurological systems) "open" to external stimulus. In human beings, one of these stimuli is meaning, as conveyed through language, performance, ritual, art, and so on.

The "placebo effect" is not an anomaly. People are simultaneously biological and cultural creatures. Biology and culture interact, and are equal partners in who and what we are. Although this is evident in many different aspects of human life, it is particularly clear when we treat one another for illness or suffering; it is, indeed, an inescapable aspect of that process. It is a fundamental part of being human. Recognizing that it is not something inherently based on deception, but on meaning, opens the possibility of many new and exciting ways of understanding human health and healing, as well as new and powerful clinical tools for healers of any kind. Turning one's eyes away from such powerful human interactions is not only short-sighted and foolish, but utterly unethical.

I began this book on a personal note telling of my experiences in South Carolina. I will finish similarly, in a personal way. People who know of my interest in these matters, primarily students, are often puzzled by how I personally respond to what I know and say about these issues. "Suppose," I have been asked many times, "That some doctor told you to have coronary artery bypass surgery. What would you do?" They know that I think a good deal of the effectiveness of such a procedure comes from its meaningful components. As with any serious and dangerous procedure,

I'd first seek a second opinion. If the second opinion were the same as the first, I would go ahead with the procedure. I would want an enthusiastic and very experienced surgeon (I know just the guy), and I would ask him to be as non-invasive as possible. I would think carefully about what the operation meant, to me, to him, to the assembled assistants – the other surgeons, the anaesthetist, the nurses – and to my family and friends. I would think carefully about the hundreds of thousands of people who are helped every year by this complex procedure, this intricate tapestry of knife and symbol. I would ask that they play Louis Armstrong recordings during the operation – loudly! – and that I be able to listen to Stan Getz and Joao Gilberto in the recovery room.

And, when I have a headache, or some aches or pains in my back or leg, I shake two ibuprofen tablets into my hand, I look at them carefully, and I say, "Guys, you are the best, the most powerful and trouble-free drugs in the world." Or something like that. Then, with a large glass of water ("Water is good, too," I think carefully to myself), down the hatch.

You know what I mean.

References

The publisher has endeavored to ensure that the URLs for external websites referred to in this book are correct and active at the time of going to press. However, the publisher has no responsibility for the websites and can make no guarantee that a site will remain live or that the content is or will remain appropriate.

Ader, Robert. 1997. The Role of Conditioning in Pharmacotherapy. In *The Placebo Effect: An Interdisciplinary Exploration.* Ed. Anne Harrington, 138–65. Cambridge, MA: Harvard University Press.

Ader, R., and N. Cohen. 1975. Behaviorally Conditioned Immunosuppression. *Psychosomatic Medicine* 37, no. 4: 333–40.

Al-Sheikh, T., K. B. Allen, S. P. Straka, D. A. Heimansohn, R. L. Fain, G. D. Hutchins, S. G. Sawada, D. P. Zipes, and E. D. Engelstein. 1999. Cardiac Sympathetic Denervation After Transmyocardial Laser Revascularization. *Circulation* 100, no. 2: 135–40.

Amanzio, M., A. Pollo, G. Maggi, and F. Benedetti. 2001. Response Variability to Analgesics: A Role for Non-Specific Activation of Endogenous Opioids. *Pain* 90, no. 3: 205–15.

American Psychiatric Association. 1994. *Diagnostic and Statistical Manual of Mental Disorders: DSM–IV.* 4th edn. Washington, DC: American Psychiatric Association.

Bailar, J. C. III. 2001. The Powerful Placebo and the Wizard of Oz. *New England Journal of Medicine* 344, no. 21: 1630–2.

Bass, M. J., C. Buck, L. Turner, G. Dickie, G. Pratt, and H. C. Robinson. 1986. The Physician's Actions and the Outcome of Illness in Family Practice. *Journal of Family Practice* 23, no. 1: 43–7.

Bates, M. S., W. T. Edwards, and K. O. Anderson. 1993. Ethnocultural Influences on Variation in Chronic Pain Perception. *Pain* 52, no. 1: 101–12.

Beecher, Henry K. 1946. Pain in Men Wounded in Battle. *The Bulletin of the US Army Medical Service* 5: 445–54.

Beers, Mark H. and Robert Berkow. 1999. *The Merck Manual.* 17th edn. Whitehouse Station, NJ: Merck & Co.

Begay, D. H., and N. C. Maryboy. 2000. The Whole Universe Is My Cathedral: A Contemporary Navajo Spiritual Synthesis. *Medical Anthropology Quarterly* 14, no. 4: 498–520.

Beinfield, Harriet, and Efrem Korngold. 1991. *Between Heaven and Earth: A Guide to Chinese Medicine.* New York: Ballantine Books.

Benedetti, F. 1996. The Opposite Effects of the Opiate Antagonist Naloxone and the Cholecystokinin Antagonist Proglumide on Placebo Analgesia. *Pain* 64, no. 3: 535–43.

———. 2000. Personal Communication (July 14, 2000).

Benedetti, F., and M. Amanzio. 1997. The Neurobiology of Placebo Analgesia: From Endogenous Opioids to Cholecystokinin. *Progress in Neurobiology* 52, no. 2: 109–25.

Benedetti, F., M. Amanzio, S. Baldi, C. Casadio, A. Cavallo, M. Mancuso, E. Ruffini, A. Oliaro, and G. Maggi. 1998. The Specific Effects of Prior Opioid Exposure on Placebo Analgesia and Placebo Respiratory Depression. *Pain* 75, no. 2–3: 313–19.

Benedetti, F., M. Amanzio, S. Baldi, C. Casadio, and G. Maggi. 1999. Inducing Placebo Respiratory Depressant Responses in Humans Via Opioid Receptors. *European Journal of Neuroscience* 11, no. 2: 625–31.

Benson, Herbert, and David P. McCallie, Jr. 1979. Angina Pectoris and the Placebo Effect. *New England Journal of Medicine* 300, no. 25: 1424–9.

Bergmann, J. F., O. Chassany, J. Gandiol, P. Deblois, J. A. Kanis, J. M. Segrestaa, C. Caulin, and R. Dahan. 1994. A Randomised Clinical Trial of the Effect of Informed Consent on the Analgesic Activity of Placebo and Naproxen in Cancer Pain. *Clinical Trials and Meta-Analysis* 29, no. 1: 41–7.

Bienenfeld, L., W. Frishman, and S. P. Glasser. 1996. The Placebo Effect in Cardiovascular Disease. *American Heart Journal* 132, no. 6: 1207–21.

Blackwell, B., S. S. Bloomfield, and C. R. Buncher. 1972. Demonstration to Medical Students of Placebo Responses and Non-Drug Factors. *Lancet* 1, no. 763: 1279–82.

Blalock, J. E. 1984. The Immune System As a Sensory Organ. *Journal of Immunology* 132, no. 3: 1067–70.

Boas, Franz. 1930. *The Religion of the Kwakiutl Indians.* Columbia University Contributions to Anthropology, vol. 10. New York: Columbia University Press.

Boissel, J. P., A. M. Philippon, E. Gauthier, J. Schbath, and J. M. Destors. 1986. Time Course of Long-Term Placebo Therapy Effects in Angina Pectoris. *European Heart Journal* 7, no. 12: 1030–6.

Bok, Sissela. 1974. The Ethics of Giving Placebos. *Scientific American* 231, no. 5: 17–23.

Booth, R. J., and K. R. Ashbridge. 1993. A Fresh Look at the Relationship Between the Psyche and Immune System: Teleological Coherence and Harmony of Purpose. *Advances, The Journal of Mind-Body Health* 9, no. 2: 4–23.

Brace, C. Loring, Harry Nelson, and Noel Korn. 1971. *Atlas of Fossil Man.* New York: Holt, Rinehart and Winston.

Braithwaite, A., and P. Cooper. Analgesic Effects of Branding in Treatment of Headaches. *British Medical Journal (Clinical Research Ed.)* 282, no. 6276: 1576–8.

Bretlau, P., J. Thomsen, M. Tos, and N. J. Johnsen. 1989. Placebo Effect in Surgery for Meniere's Disease: Nine-Year Follow-Up. *American Journal of Otology* 10, no. 4: 259–61.

Brewis, Alexandra, Karen L. Schmidt, and Mary Meyer. 2000. ADHD-Type Behavior and Harmful Dysfunction in Childhood: A Cross-Cultural Model. *American Anthropologist* 102, no. 4: 823–28.

Brody, H., and D. B. Waters. 1980. Diagnosis Is Treatment. *Journal of Family Practice* 10, no. 3: 445–9.

Brown, Norman O. 1969. *Hermes the Thief: The Evolution of a Myth.* New York: Vintage Books.

Bulkley, B. H., and R. S. Ross. 1978. Coronary-Artery Bypass Surgery: It Works, But Why? *Annals of Internal Medicine* 88, no. 6: 835–6.

Cassidy, C. M. 1998. Chinese Medicine Users in the United States. Part II: Preferred Aspects of Care. *Journal of Alternative and Complementary Medicine* 4, no. 2: 189–202.

Cattaneo, Agnelo D., Paolo E. Lucchilli, and Giorgio Filippucci. 1970. Sedative Effects of Placebo Treatment. *European Journal of Clinical Pharmacology* 3: 43–45.

CDPRG. 1980. Influence of Adherence to Treatment and Response of Cholesterol on Mortality in the Coronary Drug Project. *New England Journal of Medicine* 303, no. 18: 1038–41.

Cobb, L., G. I. Thomas, D. H. Dillard, K. A. Merendino, and R. A. Bruce. 1959. An Evaluation of Internal-Mammary Artery Ligation by a Double Blind Technic. *New England Journal of Medicine* 260, no. 22: 1115–18.

Csordas, Thomas J. 2000. Theme Issue: Ritual Healing in Navajo Society. *Medical Anthropology Quarterly* 14, no. 4: 463–602.

Dawes, Robyn M. 1994. *House of Cards: Psychology and Psychotherapy Built on Myth.* New York: The Free Press.

de Craen, A. J., D. E. Moerman, S. H. Heisterkamp, G. N. Tytgat, J. G. Tijssen, and J. Kleijnen. 1999. Placebo Effect in the Treatment of Duodenal Ulcer. *British Journal of Clinical Pharmacology* 48, no. 6: 853–60.

de Craen, A. J., P. J. Roos, A. Leonard de Vries, and J. Kleijnen. 1996. Effect of Colour of Drugs: Systematic Review of Perceived Effect of Drugs and of Their Effectiveness. *British Medical Journal* 313, no. 7072: 1624–6.

de Craen, A. J., J. G. Tijssen, J. de Gans, and J. Kleijnen. 2000. Placebo Effect in the Acute Treatment of Migraine: Subcutaneous Placebos Are Better Than Oral Placebos. *Journal of Neurology* 247, no. 3: 183–8.

de La Fuente-Fernandez, R., T. J. Ruth, V. Sossi, M. Schulzer, D. B. Calne, and A. J. Stoessl. 2001. Expectation and Dopamine Release: Mechanism of the Placebo Effect in Parkinson's Disease. *Science* 293, no. 5532: 1164–6.

Del Mar, C. B., P. P. Glasziou, and A. B. Spinks. 2000. Antibiotics for Sore Throat (Cochrane Review). *The Cochrane Library*, Issue 1.

Dimond, E. G., C. F. Kittle, and J. E. Crockett. 1960. Comparison of Internal Mammary Ligation and Sham Operation for Angina Pectoris. *American Journal of Cardiology* 5: 483–6.

Douglas, Mary. 1966. *Purity and Danger: An Analysis of the Concepts of Pollution and Taboo.* London: Routledge & Kegan Paul.

Dow, James. 1986a. *The Shaman's Touch: Otomi Indian Symbolic Healing.* Salt Lake City: University of Utah Press.

1986b. Universal Aspects of Symbolic Healing: A Theoretical Synthesis. *American Anthropologist* 88: 56–69.

Drinnan, M. J., and M. F. Marmor. 1991. Functional Visual Loss in Cambodian Refugees: A study of Cultural Factors in Ophthalmology. *European Journal of Ophthalmology* 1, no. 3: 115–18.

Dundee, J. W., R. G. Ghaly, K. M. Bill, W. N. Chestnutt, K. T. Fitzpatrick, and A. G. Lynas. 1989. Effect of Stimulation of the P6 Antiemetic Point on Postoperative Nausea and Vomiting. *British Journal of Anaesthesia* 63, no. 5: 612–8.

Edgerton, Robert B. 1971. A Traditional African Psychiatrist. *Southwestern Journal of Anthropology* 27: 259–78.

Eisenberg, D. M., R. B. Davis, S. L. Ettner, S. Appel, S. Wilkey, M. Van Rompay, and R. C. Kessler. 1998. Trends in Alternative Medicine Use in the United States, 1990–1997: Results of a Follow-Up National Survey. *Journal of the American Medical Association* 280, no. 18: 1569–75.

Ellenberg, S. S., and R. Temple. 2000. Placebo-Controlled trials and Active-Control Trials in the Evaluation of New Treatments. Part 2: Practical Issues and Specific Cases. *Annals of Internal Medicine* 133, no. 6: 464–70.

Etkin, Nina L. 1992. "Side Effects". Cultural Constructions and Reinterpretations of Western Pharmaceuticals. *Medical Anthropology Quarterly* 6, no. 2: 99–113.

Eysenck, H. J. 1952. The Effects of Psychotherapy: An Evaluation. *Journal of Consulting Psychology* 16: 319–24.

1994. The Outcome Problem in Psychotherapy: What Have We Learned? *Behaviour Research and Therapy* 32, no. 5: 477–95.

Fadem, Stephen Z. 2000. A Doctor Gets Sick. *Nephron Information Center.* Http://w.w.w.Nephron.Com/Life.Html.

Fallowfield, L. J., A. Hall, G. P. Maguire, and M. Baum. 1990. Psychological Outcomes of Different Treatment Policies in Women With Early Breast Cancer Outside a Clinical Trial. *British Medical Journal* 301, no. 6752: 575–80.

Fisher, S. 1967. The Placebo Reactor: Thesis, Antithesis, Synthesis, and Hypothesis. *Diseases of the Nervous System* 28, no. 8: 510–5.

Fisher, S., and R. L. Fisher. 1963. Placebo Response and Acquiescence. *Psychopharmacologia* 4: 298–301.

Floody, P. 2000. Personal Communication (February 28, 2000).

Gallagher, E. J., C. M. Viscoli, and R. I. Horwitz. 1993. The Relationship of Treatment Adherence to the Risk of Death After Myocardial Infarction in Women. *Journal of the American Medical Association* 270, no. 6: 742–4.

Gallucci, F., H. R. Bird, C. Berardi, V. Gallai, P. Pfanner, and A. Weinberg. 1993. Symptoms of Attention-Deficit Hyperactivity Disorder in an Italian School Sample: Findings of a Pilot Study. *Journal of the American Academy of Child and Adolescent Psychiatry* 32, no. 5: 1051–8.

Gartner, M. A., Jr. 1961. Selected Personality Differences Between Placebo Reactors and Nonreactors. *Journal of the American Osteopathic Association* 60: 377–78.

Gaw, Albert. 1993. *Culture, Ethnicity, and Mental Illness.* 1st edn. Washington, DC: American Psychiatric Press.

Geertz Clifford. 1973. Thick Description: Toward an Interpretive Theory of Culture. In *The Interpretation of Cultures.* Clifford Geertz, pp. 3–30. New York: Basic Books, Inc.

Glover, Robert P. 1957. A New Surgical Approach to the Problem of Myocardial Revascularization in Coronary Artery Disease. *Journal of Arkansas Medical Society* 54, no. 6: 223–34.

Goodman, Ellen. 2001. As Medicine Evolves, the 'Placebo Effect' Comes Undone. *Boston Globe*, May 31.

Gracely, R. H., W. R. Deeter, P. J. Wolskee, *et al.* 1979. The Effect of Naloxone on Multidimensional Scales of Postsurgical Pain in Nonsedated Patients. *Society for Neuroscience Abstracts* 5: 609.

Gracely, R. H., R. Dubner, W. R. Deeter, and P. J. Wolskee. 1985. Clinicians' Expectations Influence Placebo Analgesia. *Lancet* 1, no. 8419: 43.

Gracely, R. H., R. Dubner, P. J. Wolskee, and W. R. Deeter. 1983. Placebo and Naloxone Can Alter Post-Surgical Pain by Separate Mechanisms. *Nature* 306, no. 5940: 264–5.

Graham, N. M., C. J. Burrell, R. M. Douglas, P. Debelle, and L. Davies. 1990. Adverse Effects of Aspirin, Acetaminophen, and Ibuprofen on Immune Function, Viral Shedding, and Clinical Status in Rhinovirus-Infected Volunteers. *Journal of Infectious Diseases* 162, no. 6: 1277–82.

Grenfell, R. F., A. H. Briggs, and W. C. Holland. 1961. A Double-Blind Study of the Treatment of Hypertension. *Journal of the American Medical Association* 176: 124–8.

Grevert, P., L. H. Albert, and A. Goldstein. 1983. Partial Antagonism of Placebo Analgesia by Naloxone. *Pain* 16, no. 2: 129–43.

Gryll, S. L., and M. Katahn. 1978. Situational Factors Contributing to the Placebo Effect. *Psychopharmacology* 57: 253–61.

Gudmand-Hoyer, E., F. Frost, K. B. Jensen, E. Krag, J. Rask-Madsen, I. Rahbek, S. Rune, and H. R. Wulff. 1977. A Pragmatic Trial of Cimetidine in Duodenal Ulcer Patients. *Scandinavian Journal of Gastroenterology* 12, no. 5: 611–3.

Hahn, Robert A. 1995. *Sickness and Healing: An Anthropological Perspective.* New Haven: Yale University Press.

Harrington, Anne. 2002. "Seeing" the Placebo Effect: Historical Legacies and Present Opportunities. In *The Science of the Placebo.* Eds. Arthur Kleinman, Harold Guess, John Kusak, and Linda Engel, pp. 35–52. London: BMJ Books.

Harris, Marvin. 1985. *Good to Eat: Riddles of Food and Culture.* New York: Simon and Schuster.

Herrick, James William. 1978. Powerful Medicinal Plants in Traditional Iroquois Culture. *New York State Journal of Medicine* 78, no. 6: 979–87.

Herrick, James W., and Dean R. Snow. 1995. *Iroquois Medical Botany.* 1st edn. The Iroquois and Their Neighbors. Syracuse, NY: Syracuse University Press.

Hirsch, G. M., G. W. Thompson, R. C. Arora, K. J. Hirsch, J. A. Sullivan, and J. A. Armour. 1999. Transmyocardial Laser Revascularization Does Not

Denervate the Canine Heart. *Annals of Thoracic Surgery* 68, no. 2: 460–8; discussion 468–9.

Hogarty, G. E., and S. C. Goldberg. 1973. Drugs and Sociotherapy in the Aftercare of Schizophrenic Patients. One-Year Relapse Rates. *Archives of General Psychiatry* 28, no. 1: 54–64.

Holland, H. Z., and Peter Guerra. 1998. A Conversation With Jerome Frank: CT Interviews Pioneer in Psychotherapy. *Counseling Today,* online version. http://www.counseling.org/ctonline/archives/ct0898/frank.htm.

Horwitz, Ralph I., Catherine M. Viscoli, Lisa Berkman, Robert M. Donaldson, Sarah M. Horwitz, Carolyn J. Murray, David F. Ransohoff, and Jody Sindelar. 1990. Treatment Adherence and Risk of Death After Myocardial Infarction. *Lancet* 336: 542–45.

Houston, W. R. 1938. The Doctor Himself As a Therapeutic Agent. *Annals of Internal Medicine* 11, no. 8: 1416–25.

Hróbjartsson, A., and P. C. Gøtzsche. 2001. Is the Placebo Powerless? An Analysis of Clinical Trials Comparing Placebo With No Treatment. *New England Journal of Medicine* 344, no. 21: 1594–602.

Humphrey, Nicholas. 2002. Great Expectations: The Evolutionary Psychology of Faith-Healing and the Placebo Response. In *The Mind Made Flesh: Essays From the Frontiers of Evolution and Psychology.* Nicholas Humphrey, pp. 255–85. Oxford: Oxford University Press.

Hussain, M. Z., and A. Ahad. 1970. Tablet Colour in Anxiety States. *British Medical Journal* 3, no. 720: 466.

Idler, E. L., and S. Kasl. 1991. Health Perceptions and Survival: Do Global Evaluations of Health Status Really Predict Mortality? *Journal of Gerontology* 46, no. 2: S55–65.

Irvine, J., B. Baker, J. Smith, S. Jandciu, M. Paquette, J. Cairns, S. Connolly, R. Roberts, M. Gent, and P. Dorian. 1999. Poor Adherence to Placebo or Amiodarone Therapy Predicts Mortality: Results From the CAMIAT Study. Canadian Amiodarone Myocardial Infarction Arrhythmia Trial. *Psychosomatic Medicine* 61, no. 4: 566–75.

Johnson, A. G. 1994. Surgery As a Placebo. *Lancet* 344, no. 8930: 1140–2.

Johnson, Dirk. 1999. Many Schools Putting an End to Child's Play. *New York Times,* April 7, 1999.

Jones, James H., and Tuskegee Institute. 1981. *Bad Blood: The Tuskegee Syphilis Experiment.* New York: Free Press, London: Collier Macmillan Publishers.

Kantor, B., C. J. McKenna, J. A. Caccitolo, K. Miyauchi, G. S. Reeder, C. J. Mullany, H. V. Schaff, D. R. Holmes, Jr., and R. S. Schwartz. 1999. Transmyocardial and Percutaneous Myocardial Revascularization: Current and Future Role in the Treatment of Coronary Artery Disease. *Mayo Clinic Proceedings* 74, no. 6: 585–92.

Kaplan, G. A., and T. Camacho. 1983. Perceived Health and Mortality: A Nine-Year Follow-Up of the Human Population Laboratory Cohort. *American Journal of Epidemiology* 117, no. 3: 292–304.

Kaplan, G. A., T. E. Seeman, R. D. Cohen, L. P. Knudsen, and J. Guralnik. 1987. Mortality Among the Elderly in the Alameda County Study: Behavioral and Demographic Risk Factors. *American Journal of Public Health* 77, no. 3: 307–12.

Kewman, D., and A. H. Roberts. 1980. Skin Temperature Biofeedback and Migraine Headaches. A Double-Blind Study. *Biofeedback and Self Regulation* 5, no. 3: 327–45.

Kirmayer, L. J., and A. Young. 1998. Culture and Somatization: Clinical, Epidemiological, and Ethnographic Perspectives. *Psychosomatic Medicine* 60, no. 4: 420–30.

Kirsch, I., and L. J. Weixel. 1988. Double-Blind Versus Deceptive Administration of a Placebo. *Behavioral Neuroscience* 102, no. 2: 319–23.

Kitchell, J. R., R. P. Glover, and R. H. Kyle. 1958. Bilateral Internal Mammary Artery Ligation for Angina Pectoris: Preliminary Clinical Considerations. *American Journal of Cardiology* 1: 46–50.

Kleinman, Arthur, M. D. 1988. *Rethinking Psychiatry: From Cultural Category to Personal Experience.* New York: The Free Press.

Kluckhohn, Cylde, and Leland C. Wyman. 1940. An Introduction to Navaho Chant Practice. *Memoirs of the American Anthropological Association* 53: 1–204.

Knipschild, P., P. Leffers, and A. R. Feinstein. 1991. The Qualification Period. *Journal of Clinical Epidemiology* 44, no. 6: 461–4.

Knipschild, P., P. Leffers, and A. R. Feinstein. 1992. Value for the Money. *Journal of Clinical Epidemiology* 45: 564–65.

Lambert, R., J. P. Bader, J. J. Bernier, J. Bertrand, C. Betourne, J. Gastard, C. Laverdant, A. Ribet, J. Sahel, and J. Toulet. 1977. Treatment of Duodenal and Gastric Ulcer with Cimetidine. A Multicenter Double-Blind Trial. *Gastroenterologie Clinique Et Biologique* 1, no. 11: 855–60.

Landman, J. T., and R. M. Dawes. 1982. Psychotherapy Outcome. Smith and Glass' Conclusions Stand Up Under Scrutiny. *American Psychologist* 37, no. 5: 504–16.

Landolfo, C. K., K. P. Landolfo, G. C. Hughes, E. R. Coleman, R. B. Coleman, and J. E. Lowe. 1999. Intermediate-Term Clinical Outcome Following Transmyocardial Laser Revascularization in Patients With Refractory Angina Pectoris. *Circulation* 100, no. 19, Supplement II: 128–33.

Landray, M. J., and G. Y. Lip. 1999. White Coat Hypertension: A Recognised Syndrome With Uncertain Implications. *Journal of Human Hypertension* 13, no. 1: 5–8.

Lang, J. M. 1992. No Free Lunch. *Journal of Clinical Epidemiology* 45: 563–65.

Lange, R. A., and L. D. Hillis. 1999. Transmyocardial Laser Revascularization. *New England Journal of Medicine* 341, no. 14: 1075–6.

Lanza, F., J. Goff, C. Scowcroft, D. Jennings, and P. Greski-Rose. 1994. Double-Blind Comparison of Lansoprazole, Ranitidine, and Placebo in the Treatment of Acute Duodenal Ulcer. Lansoprazole Study Group. *American Journal of Gastroenterology* 89, no. 8: 1191–200.

Laporte, J. R., and A. Figueras. 1994. Placebo Effects in Psychiatry. *Lancet* 344, no. 8931: 1206–9.

Lasagna, L. 1986. The Placebo Effect. *Journal of Allergy Clinical Immunology* 78, no. 1, Part 2: 161–5.

Lebra, William P. 1976. *Culture-Bound Syndromes, Ethnopsychiatry, and Alternate*

Therapies. Mental Health Research in Asia and the Pacific, vol. 4. Honolulu: University Press of Hawaii.

Leon, Martin. 2000. DMR in Regeneration of Endomyocardial Channels Trial (DIRECT). *American College of Cardiology* http://www.acc.org/education/online/trials/aha00/direct.htm.

Leon, Martin B., Donald S. Baim, Jeffery W. Moses, Roger J. Laham, and William Knopf. 2000. A Randomized Blinded Clinical Trial Comparing Percutaneous Laser Myocardial Revascularization (Using Biosnese LV Mapping) Vs. Placebo in Patients With Refractory Coronary Ischemia. Paper Presented on American College of Cardiology website, http://www.ac.org/education/online/trials/aha00/direct.htm.

Leroi-Gourhan, Arlette. 1975. The Flowers Found with Shanidar IV, a Neanderthal Burial in Iraq. *Science* 190: 562–64.

1998. Shanidar Et Ses Fleurs. *Paléorient* 24, no. 2: 79–88.

Leslie, Alan. 1954. Ethics and Practice of Placebo Therapy. *American Journal of Medicine* 16: 854–56.

Leung, P. W., S. L. Luk, T. P. Ho, E. Taylor, F. L. Mak, and J. Bacon-Shone. 1996. The Diagnosis and Prevalence of Hyperactivity in Chinese Schoolboys. *British Journal of Psychiatry* 168, no. 4: 486–96.

Levi-Strauss, Claude. 1967a. The Effectiveness of Symbols. In *Structural Anthropology*. Levi-Strauss, 180–201. Garden City, NY: Anchor Books.

1967b. The Sorcerer and His Magic. In *Structural Anthropology*. Levi-Strauss, 160–80. Garden City, NY: Anchor Books.

Levine, J. D., N. C. Gordon, and H. L. Fields. 1978. The Mechanism of Placebo Analgesia. *Lancet* 2, no. 8091: 654–7.

Liberman, R. P. 1967. The Elusive Placebo Reactor. *Neuro-Psycho-Pharmacology: Proceedings of the Fifth International Congress of the Collegium Internationale Neuro-Psycho-Pharmacologicum*, Chief Editor H. Brill, 557–66. Amsterdam: Excerpta Medica Foundation.

Linde, C., F. Gadler, L. Kappenberger, and L. Ryden. 1999. Placebo Effect of Pacemaker Implantation in Obstructive Hypertrophic Cardiomyopathy. PIC Study Group. Pacing In Cardiomyopathy. *American Journal of Cardiology* 83, no. 6: 903–7.

Lock, Margaret M. 1986a. Ambiguities of Aging: Japanese Experience and Perceptions of Menopause. *Culture, Medicine and Psychiatry* 10: 23–46.

1986b. Introduction to Anthropological Approaches to Menopause. *Culture, Medicine, and Psychiatry* 10, no. 1: 1–7.

1993. The Politics of Mid-Life and Menopause: Ideologies for the Second Sex in North America and Japan. *Knowledge, Power and Practice: The Anthropology of Medicine and Everyday Life*. Eds. Shirley Lindenbaum and Margaret Lock, 330–63. Berkeley, CA: University of California Press.

Luborsky, L., B. Singer, and L. Luborsky. 1975. Comparative Studies of Psychotherapies. Is It True that "Everyone Has Won and All Must Have Prizes"? *Archives of General Psychiatry* 32, no. 8: 995–1008.

Lucchelli, P. E., A. D. Cattaneo, and J. Zattoni. 1978. Effect of Capsule Colour and Order of Administration of Hypnotic Treatments. *European Journal of Clinical Pharmacology* 13, no. 2: 153–5.

Malchow, H., K. F. Sewing, M. Albinus, B. Horn, H. Schomerus, and W. Dolle. 1978. [In-patient Treatment of Peptic Ulcer with Cimetidine. I. Effect on Duodenal Ulcer Healing (author's translation)]. *Deutsche Medizinische Wochenschrift* 103, no. 4: 149–52.

Maretzki, T. W. 1987. The Kur in West Germany as an Interface Between Naturopathic and Allopathic Ideologies. *Social Science and Medicine* 24, no. 12: 1061–8.

MCATT. 1982. Untreated Mild Hypertension. *Lancet* 1: 185–91.

McGrath, P. A. 1994. Psychological Aspects of Pain Perception. *Archives of Oral Biology* 39, Supplement: 55S–62S.

McGrew, W. C., and C. E. G. Tutin. 1972. Chimpanzee Dentistry. *Journal of the American Dental Association* 85: 1198–204.

Meade, Richard H. 1961. *A History of Thoracic Surgery.* Springfield, IL: C.C. Thomas.

Medical Outcomes Trust, and Ware, John E. Jr. 2000. "The SF-36 Health Survey." Web page. Available at http://www.qmetric.com/products/assessments/sf36/SF-36.pdf, July, 2000.

Melzack, R., and P. D. Wall. 1965. Pain Mechanisms: A New Theory. *Science* 150, no. 699: 971–9.

Miner, Horace. 1956. Body Ritual of the Nacirema. *American Anthropologist* 58: 503–7.

Moerman, Daniel E. 1979. Anthropology of Symbolic Healing. *Current Anthropology* 20, no. 1: 59–80.

1982. *Geraniums for the Iroquois: A Field Guide to American Indian Medicinal Plants.* Algonac, MI: Reference Publications.

1983. Physiology and Symbols: The Anthropological Implications of the Placebo Effect. In *The Anthropology of Medicine: From Culture to Method.* 1st edn. Eds. Lola Romanucci-Ross, Daniel E. Moerman, and Laurence R. Tancredi, pp. 156–67. Westport, CT: Bergin and Garvey.

1989. Poisoned Apples and Honeysuckles: The Medicinal Plants of Native America. *Medical Anthropology Quarterly* 3: 52–61.

1998a. Medical Romanticism and the Sources of Medical Practice. *Complementary Therapies in Medicine* 6: 198–202.

1998b. *Native American Ethnobotany.* Portland, OR: Timber Press.

2000. Cultural Variations in the Placebo Effect: Ulcers, Anxiety, and Blood Pressure. *Medical Anthropology Quarterly* 14, no. 1: 1–22.

Montgomery, Guy, and Irving Kirsch. 1996. Mechanisms of Placebo Pain Reduction: An Empirical Investigation. *Psychological Science* 7, no. 3: 174–6.

Morris, David B. 1997. Placebo, Pain, and Belief: A Biocultural Model. In *The Placebo Effect: An Interdisciplinary Exploration.* Ed. Anne Harrington, pp. 187–207. Cambridge, MA: Harvard University Press.

Morris, J., and G. T. Royle. 1988. Offering Patients a Choice of Surgery for Early Breast Cancer: A Reduction in Anxiety and Depression in Patients and Their Husbands. *Social Science and Medicine* 26, no. 6: 583–5.

Moseley, J. B. Jr., N. P. Wray, D. Kuykendall, K. Willis, and G. Landon. 1996. Arthroscopic Treatment of Osteoarthritis of the Knee: A Prospective, Randomized, Placebo-Controlled Trial. Results of a Pilot Study. *American Journal of Sports Medicine* 24, no. 1: 28–34.

Mossey, J. M., and E. Shapiro. 1982. Self-Rated Health: A Predictor of Mortality Among the Elderly. *American Journal of Public Health* 72, no. 8: 800–8.

Mouridsen, S. E., and S. Nielsen. 1990. Reversible Somatotropin Deficiency (Psychosocial Dwarfism) Presenting As Conduct Disorder and Growth Hormone Deficiency. *Development Medicine and Child Neurology* 32, no. 12: 1093–8.

Muller, B. P. 1965. Personality of Placebo Reactors and Nonreactors. *Diseases of the Nervous System* 26: 58–61.

Murkin, J. M., W. D. Boyd, S. Ganapathy, S. J. Adams, and R. C. Peterson. 1999. Beating Heart Surgery: Why Expect Less Central Nervous System Morbidity? *Annals of Thoracic Surgery* 68, no. 4: 1498–501.

O'Brien, E. 1999. White Coat Hypertension: How Should It Be Diagnosed? *Journal of Human Hypertension* 13, no. 12: 801–2.

Parloff, M. B. 1986. Frank's "Common Elements" in Psychotherapy: Nonspecific Factors and Placebos. *American Journal of Orthopsychiatry* 56, no. 4: 521–30.

Payer, Lynn. 1996. *Medicine and Culture.* New York: Henry Holt and Company.

Pennebaker, J. W. 1990. *Opening Up. The Healing Power of Confiding in Others.* 1st edn. New York: Wm. Morrow & Co.

Pennebaker, J. W., S. D. Barger, and J. Tiebout. 1989. Disclosure of Traumas and Health Among Holocaust Survivors. *Psychosomatic Medicine* 51, no. 5: 577–89.

Petrie, K. J., R. J. Booth, J. W. Pennebaker, K. P. Davison, and M. G. Thomas. 1995. Disclosure of Trauma and Immune Response to a Hepatitis B Vaccination Program. *Journal of Consulting and Clinical Psychology* 63, no. 5: 787–92.

Pittman, Q. J., W. L. Veale, and K. E. Cooper. 1976. Observations on the Effect of Salicylate in Fever and the Regulation of Body Temperature Against Cold. *Canadian Journal of Physiology and Pharmacology* 54, no. 2: 101–6.

Pizzo, P. A., K. J. Robichaud, B. K. Edwards, C. Schumaker, B. S. Kramer, and A. Johnson. 1983. Oral Antibiotic Prophylaxis in Patients With Cancer: A Double-Blind Randomized Placebo-Controlled Trial. *Journal of Pediatrics* 102, no. 1: 125–33.

Price, D. D. 2001. Assessing Placebo Effects Without Placebo Groups: An Untapped Possibility? *Pain* 90, no. 3: 201–3.

Rothman, K. J. 1996. Placebo Mania. *British Medical Journal* 313, no. 7048: 3–4.

Rozee, P. and G. Van Boemel. 1989. The Psychological Effects of War Trauma and Abuse on Older Cambodian Refugee Women. *Women and Therapy* 8: 23–50.

Sahlins, Marshall. 1976. *The Use and Abuse of Biology: An Anthropological Critique of Sociobiology.* Ann Arbor: University of Michigan Press.

1978. *Culture and Practical Reason.* Chicago, IL: University of Chicago Press.

Salgado, J. A., C. A. de Oliveira, G. F. Lima Jr., and L. de Paula Castro. 1981. Endoscopic Findings after Antacid, Cimetidine and Placebo for Peptic Ulcer – Importance of Staging the Lesions. *Arquivos De Gastroenterologia* 18, no. 2: 51–3.

Salinger, J. D. 1955. *Franny and Zooey.* Boston: Little, Brown and Company.

Sallis, R. E., and L. W. Buckalew. 1984. Relation of Capsule Color and Perceived Potency. *Perceptual and Motor Skills* 58, no. 3: 897–8.

Schapira, K., H. A. McClelland, N. R. Griffiths, and D. J. Newell. 1970. Study on the Effects of Tablet Colour in the Treatment of Anxiety States. *British Medical Journal* 1, no. 707: 446–9.

Schoenberger, J. A., and D. J. Wilson. 1986. Once-Daily Treatment of Essential Hypertension with Captopril. *Journal of Clinical Hypertension* 2, no. 4: 379–87.

Shapiro, Arthur K. 1964. Etiological Factors in Placebo Effect. *Journal of the American Medical Association* 187, no. 10: 712–15.

Shapiro, Arthur K., and Elaine Shapiro. 1997. *The Powerful Placebo From Ancient Priest to Modern Physician*. Baltimore, MD: Johns Hopkins University Press.

Sheldon, Ben C., and Simon Verhulst. 1996. Ecological Immunology: Costly Parasite Defences and Trade-Offs in Evolutionary Ecology. *Trends in Ecology and Evolution* 11: 317–21.

Silko, Leslie Marmon. 1988. *Ceremony*. New York: Viking Penguin Inc.

Simons, Ronald C., and Charles C. Hughes. 1985. *The Culture-Bound Syndromes: Folk Illnesses of Psychiatric and Anthropological Interest*. Culture, Illness, and Healing. Dordrecht, Boston, Hingham, MA: D. Reidel.

Smith, M. L., and G. V. Glass. 1977. Meta-Analysis of Psychotherapy Outcome Studies. *American Psychologist* 32, no. 9: 752–60.

Snow, Loudell F. 1993. *Walkin' Over Medicine*. Boulder, CO: Westview Press.

Solecki, Ralph S. 1975. Shanidar IV, a Neanderthal Flower Burial in Northern Iraq. *Science* 190: 880–1.

Sontag, Susan. 1977. *Illness as Metaphor*. New York: Farrar, Straus and Giroux. 1988. *Aids and Its Metaphors*. New York: Farrar, Straus and Giroux.

Spangfort, E. V. 1972. The Lumbar Disc Herniation. A Computer-Aided Analysis of 2,504 Operations. *Acta Orthopaedica Scandinavica Supplementum* 142: 1–95.

Starfield, B., C. Wray, K. Hess, R. Gross, P. S. Birk, and B. C. D'Lugoff. 1981. The Influence of Patient–Practitioner Agreement on Outcome of Care. *American Journal of Public Health* 71, no. 2: 127–31.

Sternbach, Richard, and Bernard Tursky. 1965. Ethnic Differences Among Housewives in Psychophysical and Skin Potential Responses to Electric Shock. *Psychophysiology* 1: 241–46.

Stewart, M. A. 1995. Effective Physician–Patient Communication and Health Outcomes: A Review. *CMAJ* 152, no. 9: 1423–33.

Straus, B., J. Eisenberg, and J. Gennis. 1955. Hypnotic Effects of an Antihistamine–Methapyrilene Hydrochloride. *Annals of Internal Medicine* 42: 574.

Strupp, H. H. 1986. The Nonspecific Hypothesis of Therapeutic Effectiveness: A Current Assessment. *American Journal of Orthopsychiatry* 56, no. 4: 513–20.

Strupp, H. H., and S. W. Hadley. 1979. Specific Vs. Nonspecific Factors in Psychotherapy. A Controlled Study of Outcome. *Archives of General Psychiatry* 36, no. 10: 1125–36.

Svensson, E., L. Råberg, C. Koch, and D. Hasselquist. 1998. Energetic Stress, Imunosuppression and the Costs of an Antibody Response. *Functional Ecology* 12: 912–19.

Talbot, Margaret. 2000. The Placebo Prescription. *New York Times Magazine*. January 9. 34–39, 44, 58–60.

Talley, P. F., H. H. Strupp, and L. C. Morey. 1990. Matchmaking in Psychotherapy: Patient–Therapist Dimensions and Their Impact on Outcome. *Journal of Consulting and Clinical Psychology* 58, no. 2: 182–8.

Temple, R., and S. S. Ellenberg. 2000. Placebo-Controlled Trials and Active-Control Trials in the Evaluation of New Treatments. Part 1: Ethical and Scientific Issues. *Annals of Internal Medicine* 133, no. 6: 455–63.

Thomas, K. B. 1987. General Practice Consultations: Is There Any Point in Being Positive? *British Medical Journal* 294, no. 6581: 1200–2.

Thomsen, J., P. Bretlau, M. Tos, and N. J. Johnsen. 1981. Placebo Effect in Surgery for Meniere's Disease. A Double-Blind, Placebo-Controlled Study on Endolymphatic Sac Shunt Surgery. *Archives of Otolaryngology* 107, no. 5: 271–7.

Trivedi, M. H., and H. Rush. 1994. Does a Placebo Run-in or a Placebo Treatment Cell Affect the Efficacy of Antidepressant Medications? *Neuropsychopharmacology* 11, no. 1: 33–43.

Turner, J. A., R. A. Deyo, J. D. Loeser, M. Von Korff, and W. E. Fordyce. 1994. The Importance of Placebo Effects in Pain Treatment and Research. *Journal of the American Medical Association* 271, no. 20: 1609–14.

Tursky, Bernard, and Richard A. Sternbach. 1967. Further Physiological Correlates of Ethnic Differences in Responses to Shock. *Psychophysiology*, no. 67–74.

Uhlenhuth, E. H., K. Rickels, S. Fisher, L. C. Park, R. S. Lipman, and J. Mock. 1966. Drug, Doctor's Verbal Attitude and Clinic Setting in Symptomatic Response to Pharmacotherapy. *Psychopharmacology* 9: 392–418.

Ulrich, R. S. 1984. View Through a Window May Influence Recovery From Surgery. *Science* 224, no. 4647: 420–1.

Vaccarino, A. L., and A. J. Kastin. 2000. Endogenous Opiates: 1999. *Peptides* 21, no. 12: 1975–2034.

Valdes, M., B. D. McCallister, D. R. McConahay, W. A. Reed, D. A. Killen, and M. Arnold. 1979. "Sham Operation" Revisited: A Comparison of Complete Vs. Unsuccessful Coronary Artery Bypass. *American Journal of Cardiology* 43: 382.

Vickers, A. J. 1996. Can Acupuncture Have Specific Effects on Health? A Systematic Review of Acupuncture Antiemesis Trials. *Journal of the Royal Society of Medicine* 89, no. 6: 303–11.

Walike, B. C., and B. Meyer. 1966. Relation Between Placebo Reactivity and Selected Personality Factors. *Nursing Research.* 15: 119–23.

Wall, P. D. 1993. Pain and the Placebo Response. *Ciba Foundation Symposium* 174: 187–211; discussion 212–6.

Watkins, A. D. 1995. Perceptions, Emotions and Immunity: An Integrated Homeostatic Network. *Quarterly Journal of Medicine* 88, no. 4: 283–94.

Welling, D. B., and H. N. Nagaraja. 2000. Endolymphatic Mastoid Shunt: A Re-evaluation of Efficacy. *Otolaryngology – Head and Neck Surgery* 122, no. 3: 340–5.

White, J. M. 1999. Effects of Relaxing Music on Cardiac Autonomic Balance and Anxiety After Acute Myocardial Infarction. *American Journal of Critical Care* 8, no. 4: 220–30.

Whitehorn, John C., and Barbara J. Betz. 1960. Further Studies of the Doctor As a Crucial Variable in the Outcome of Treatment With Schizophrenic Patients. *American Journal of Psychiatry* 117, no. 3: 215–23.

Wickramasekera, I. 1980. A Conditioned Response Model of the Placebo Effect Predictions From the Model. *Biofeedback and Self Regulation* 5, no. 1: 5–18.

Wierzbicka, Anna. 1989. Soul and Mind: Linguistic Evidence for Ethnopsychology and Cultural History. *American Anthropologist* 91: 41–58.

Wolff, B. Berthold, and Sarah Langley. 1968. Cultural Factors and the Response to Pain. *American Anthropologist* 70, no. 3: 494–501.

World Health Organization. 1992. *ICD–10 International Statistical Classification of Diseases and Related Health Problems*. 10th edn. Geneva: World Health Organization.

World Medical Association. "Welcome to the World Medical Association." Web page, available at http://www.wma.net/.

Wyman, Leland Clifton. 1970. *Blessingway. With Three Versions of the Myth Recorded and Translated From the Navajo by Berard Haile*. Translator Berard Haile. Tucson: University of Arizona Press.

Zborowski, Mark. 1952. Cultural Components in Responses to Pain. *Journal of Social Issues* 8: 16–30.

1969. *People in Pain*. 1st edn. The Jossey-Bass Behavioral Science Series. San Francisco: Jossey-Bass.

Zohar, A. H., G. Ratzoni, D. L. Pauls, A. Apter, A. Bleich, S. Kron, M. Rappaport, A. Weizman, and D. J. Cohen. 1992. An Epidemiological Study of Obsessive-Compulsive Disorder and Related Disorders in Israeli Adolescents. *Journal of the American Academy of Child and Adolescent Psychiatry* 31, no. 6: 1057–61.

Index